Clinical and Molecular Aspects of Cardiomyopathies: On the Road from Gene to Therapy

Editors

SHARLENE M. DAY
PERRY M. ELLIOTT
GIUSEPPE LIMONGELLI

HEART FAILURE CLINICS

www.heartfailure.theclinics.com

Consulting Editor
EDUARDO BOSSONE

Founding Editor
JAGAT NARULA

April 2018 • Volume 14 • Number 2

ELSEVIER

1600 John F. Kennedy Boulevard • Suite 1800 • Philadelphia, Pennsylvania, 19103-2899

http://www.theclinics.com

HEART FAILURE CLINICS Volume 14, Number 2
April 2018 ISSN 1551-7136, ISBN-13: 978-0-323-61046-9

Editor: Stacy Eastman
Developmental Editor: Laura Fisher

Heart Failure Clinics (ISSN 1551-7136) is published quarterly by Elsevier Inc., 360 Park Avenue South, New York, NY 10010-1710. Months of publication are January, April, July, and October. Business and editorial offices: 1600 John F. Kennedy Boulevard, Suite 1800, Philadelphia, PA 19103-2899. Periodicals postage paid at New York, NY, and additional mailing offices. Subscription prices are USD 252.00 per year for US individuals, USD 471.00 per year for US institutions, USD 100.00 per year for US students and residents, USD 294.00 per year for Canadian individuals, USD 545.00 per year for Canadian institutions, USD 309.00 per year for international individuals, USD 545.00 per year for international institutions, and USD 100.00 per year for Canadian and foreign students/residents. To receive student and resident rate, orders must be accompanied by name of affiliated institution, date of term, and the *signature* of program/residency coordinator on institution letterhead. Orders will be billed at individual rate until proof of status is received. Foreign air speed delivery is included in all *Clinics* subscription prices. All prices are subject to change without notice. **POSTMASTER:** Send address changes to *Heart Failure Clinics*, Elsevier Health Sciences Division, Subscription Customer Service, 3251 Riverport Lane, Maryland Heights, MO 63043. **Customer Service: 1-800-654-2452 (US and Canada). From outside of the US and Canada, call 314-447-8871. Fax: 314-447-8029. For print support, E-mail: JournalsCustomerService-usa@elsevier.com. For online support, E-mail: JournalsOnlineSupport-usa@elsevier.com.**

Reprints. For copies of 100 or more of articles in this publication, please contact the Commercial Reprints Department, Elsevier Inc., 360 Park Avenue South, New York, NY 10010-1710. Tel.: 212-633-3874; Fax: 212-633-3820; E-mail: reprints@elsevier.com.

Heart Failure Clinics is covered in *MEDLINE/PubMed (Index Medicus)*.

Contributors

CONSULTING EDITOR

EDUARDO BOSSONE, MD, PhD, FESC, FACC
"Cava de' Tirreni and Amalfi Coast," Division of Cardiology, Heart Department, University Hospital; Cardiology Division, University of Salerno, Salerno, Italy

EDITORS

SHARLENE M. DAY, MD
Associate Professor, Department of Internal Medicine, Division of Cardiovascular Medicine, Department of Molecular and Integrative Physiology; Director, Program for Inherited Cardiomyopathies, University of Michigan, Ann Arbor, Michigan, USA

PERRY M. ELLIOTT, MBBS, MD
Professor, Chair of Cardiovascular Medicine, University College London; Head, Clinical Research, UCL Institute of Cardiovascular Science; Consultant Cardiologist, Barts Heart Centre, London, United Kingdom

GIUSEPPE LIMONGELLI, MD, PhD
Associate Professor, Department of Cardiothoracic Sciences, Università della Campania "Luigi Vanvitelli"; Head, Cardiovascular Rare Disease Unit, Cardiomyopathies and Heart Failure Unit, Monaldi Hospital, AORN Colli, Naples, Italy; Honorary Senior Lecturer, UCL Institute of Cardiovascular Science, London, United Kingdom

AUTHORS

RACHELE ADORISIO, MD
Department of Pediatric Cardiology and Cardiac Surgery, Bambino Gesù Children's Hospital and Research Institute, Rome, Italy

ENRICO AMMIRATI, MD, PhD
"De Gasperis" Cardio Center and Transplant Center, ASST Grande Ospedale Metropolitano Niguarda, Milan, Italy

GOURG ATTEYA, MD
SUNY Downstate Medical Center, Yale School of Medicine, New Haven, Connecticut, USA

ANWAR BABAN, MD, PhD
Department of Pediatric Cardiology and Cardiac Surgery, Bambino Gesù Children's Hospital and Research Institute, Rome, Italy

RICHARD D. BAGNALL, PhD
Senior Research Officer, Agnes Ginges Centre for Molecular Cardiology, Centenary Institute; Conjoint Senior Lecturer, Sydney Medical School, University of Sydney, New South Wales, Australia

CRISTINA BASSO, MD, PhD
Department of Cardiac, Thoracic, and Vascular
Sciences, University of Padova Medical
School, Padova, Italy

BARBARA BAUCE, MD, PhD
Department of Cardiac, Thoracic, and Vascular
Sciences, University of Padova Medical
School, Padova, Italy

**EDUARDO BOSSONE, MD, PhD, FESC,
FACC**
"Cava de' Tirreni and Amalfi Coast," Division of
Cardiology, Heart Department, University
Hospital; Cardiology Division, University of
Salerno, Salerno, Italy

GIULIO CALCAGNI, MD, PhD
Department of Pediatric Cardiology and
Cardiac Surgery, Bambino Gesù Children's
Hospital and Research Institute, Rome, Italy

RAFFAELE COPPINI, MD, PhD
Department NeuroFarBa, University of
Florence, Florence, Italy

DOMENICO CORRADO, MD, PhD
Department of Cardiac, Thoracic, and Vascular
Sciences, University of Padova Medical
School, Padova, Italy

SHARLENE M. DAY, MD
Associate Professor, Department of Internal
Medicine, Division of Cardiovascular Medicine,
Department of Molecular and Integrative
Physiology; Director, Program for Inherited
Cardiomyopathies, University of Michigan,
Ann Arbor, Michigan, USA

MARIA CRISTINA DIGILIO, MD
Genetics and Rare Diseases Research
Division, Bambino Gesù Children's Hospital
and Research Institute, Rome, Italy

FABRIZIO DRAGO, MD
Department of Pediatric Cardiology and
Cardiac Surgery, Bambino Gesù Children's
Hospital and Research Institute, Rome, Italy

PERRY M. ELLIOTT, MBBS, MD
Professor, Chair of Cardiovascular
Medicine, University College London; Head,
Clinical Research, UCL Institute of
Cardiovascular Science, Consultant
Cardiologist, Barts Heart Centre, London,
United Kingdom

AMANDA C. GARFINKEL, BA
Medical Student, Sarnoff Cardiovascular
Research Fellow, Department of Genetics,
Harvard Medical School, Boston,
Massachusetts, USA

BRUCE D. GELB, MD
Department of Pediatrics and Genetics and
Genomic Sciences, Icahn School of Medicine
at Mount Sinai, The Mindich Child Health and
Development Institute, New York, New York,
USA

GIORGIA GRUTTER, MD
Department of Pediatric Cardiology
and Cardiac Surgery, Bambino Gesù
Children's Hospital and Research Institute,
Rome, Italy

JODIE INGLES, PhD, MPH
Senior Research Officer, Agnes Ginges Centre
for Molecular Cardiology, Centenary Institute;
Senior Lecturer, Sydney Medical School,
University of Sydney; Cardiac Genetic
Counsellor, Department of Cardiology, Royal
Prince Alfred Hospital, Sydney, New South
Wales, Australia

JUAN PABLO KASKI, MD
Centre for Inherited Cardiovascular Diseases,
Great Ormond Street Hospital, UCL Institute of
Cardiovascular Science, London, United
Kingdom

RACHEL LAMPERT, MD
Professor of Medicine, Yale School of
Medicine, New Haven, Connecticut, USA

SARAH J. LEHMAN, PhD
Post-Doctoral Research Associate,
Department of Physiological
Sciences, University of Arizona, Tucson,
Arizona, USA

GIUSEPPE LIMONGELLI, MD, PhD
Associate Professor, Department of
Cardiothoracic Sciences, Università della
Campania "Luigi Vanvitelli"; Head,
Cardiovascular Rare Disease Unit,
Cardiomyopathies and Heart Failure Unit,
Monaldi Hospital, AORN Colli, Naples, Italy;
Honorary Senior Lecturer, UCL Institute of
Cardiovascular Science, London, United
Kingdom

MELISSA L. LYNN, PhD
Post-Doctoral Research Associate,
Department of Medicine, University of Arizona,
Tucson, Arizona, USA

BRUNO MARINO, MD
Pediatric Cardiology, Department of
Pediatrics, Sapienza University, Rome, Italy

SIMONE MARTINELLI, PhD
Department of Oncology and Molecular
Medicine, Istituto Superiore di Sanità, Rome,
Italy

DANIELE MASARONE, MD, PhD
Cardiomyopathies and Heart Failure Unit,
Monaldi Hospital, Naples, Italy

NICCOLÒ MAURIZI, MD
Cardiomyopathy Unit, Careggi University
Hospital; Department of Clinical and
Experimental Medicine, University of Florence,
Florence, Italy

ELIZABETH M. McNALLY, MD, PhD
Center for Genetic Medicine, Northwestern
University Feinberg School of Medicine,
Chicago, Illinois, USA

LUISA MESTRONI, MD
Adult Medical Genetics Program,
Cardiovascular Institute, University of
Colorado Anschutz, Aurora, Colorado, USA

AMELIA MORRONE, PhD
Paediatric Neurology Unit and Laboratories,
Neuroscience Department, Meyer Children's
Hospital, Florence, Italy

JOYCE C. OHIRI, BS
Center for Genetic Medicine, Northwestern
University Feinberg School of Medicine,
Chicago, Illinois, USA

IACOPO OLIVOTTO, MD
Cardiomyopathy Unit, Careggi University
Hospital, Florence, Italy

GIUSEPPE PACILEO, MD
Cardiomyopathies and Heart Failure Unit,
Monaldi Hospital, AORN Colli, Naples, Italy

KALLIOPI PILICHOU, PhD
Department of Cardiac, Thoracic, and Vascular
Sciences, University of Padova Medical
School, Padova, Italy

CHRISTINE E. SEIDMAN, MD
Departments of Medicine and Genetics,
Brigham and Women's Hospital, Harvard
Medical School, Boston, Massachusetts;
Howard Hughes Medical Institute, Chevy
Chase, Maryland, USA

JONATHAN G. SEIDMAN, PhD
Department of Genetics, Harvard Medical
School, Boston, Massachusetts, USA

**CHRISTOPHER SEMSARIAN, MBBS, PhD,
MPH**
Head, Agnes Ginges Centre for Molecular
Cardiology, Centenary Institute; Professor,
Sydney Medical School, University of Sydney;
Cardiologist, Department of Cardiology, Royal
Prince Alfred Hospital, Sydney, New South
Wales, Australia

MARY E. SWEET, BA
Adult Medical Genetics Program,
Cardiovascular Institute, University of
Colorado Anschutz, Aurora, Colorado, USA

JIL C. TARDIFF, MD, PhD
Professor, Department of Medicine, University
of Arizona, Tucson, Arizona, USA

MARCO TARTAGLIA, PhD
Genetics and Rare Diseases Research
Division, Bambino Gesù Children's Hospital
and Research Institute, Rome, Italy

MATTHEW R.G. TAYLOR, MD, PhD
Adult Medical Genetics Program,
Cardiovascular Institute, University of
Colorado Anschutz, Aurora, Colorado, USA

GAETANO THIENE, MD
Department of Cardiac, Thoracic, and Vascular
Sciences, University of Padova Medical
School, Padova, Italy

PAOLO VERSACCI, MD, PhD
Pediatric Cardiology, Department of Pediatrics,
Sapienza, Italy University, Rome, Italy

Contents

Cardiomyopathies (CMPs) are an increasingly recognized cause of heart failure and sudden death, particularly in young patients. Since their original description, major advances were achieved in the phenotype knowledge, natural history, and nosography of CMPs leading to different classification systems and therapies. However, a deeper knowledge of different causes, genotype-phenotype link, and natural history in different disease stages (preclinical, overt disease, and end-stage disease) according to a recognized standard of care (ie, international guidelines) is needed. Clinical registries can fill gaps in our knowledge regarding the uncovered issues on cause, clinical course, and management of CMPs.

Cardiac genetic testing for inherited cardiomyopathies has become a routine aspect of care. Advances in genetic testing technologies have made testing more comprehensive and affordable. With this increase comes greater understanding of the genetic basis of these diseases, but also shines a light on the challenges. Ability to ascertain whether a rare variant is causative of disease is problematic. A genetic diagnosis in a family can offer an invaluable tool for cascade genetic testing of at-risk relatives and avenues for reproductive testing options. A careful approach to cardiac genetic testing that recognizes where there is potential for harm ensures the best possible outcomes for families.

Sarcomere cardiomyopathies are genetic diseases that perturb contractile function and lead to hypertrophic or dilated myocardial remodeling. Identification of preclinical mutation carriers has yielded insights into the earliest biomechanical defects that link pathogenic variants to cardiac dysfunction. Understanding this early molecular pathophysiology can illuminate modifiable pathways to reduce the emergence of overt cardiomyopathy and curb adverse outcomes. Here, the authors review current understandings of how human hypertrophic cardiomyopathy–linked and hypertrophic dilated cardiomyopathy–linked mutations disrupt the normal structure and function of the sarcomere.

This article focuses on 3 "bins" that comprise sets of biophysical derangements elicited by cardiomyopathy-associated mutations in the myofilament. Current therapies focus on symptom palliation and do not address the disease at its core. We and others have proposed that a more nuanced classification could lead to direct interventions based on early dysregulation changing the trajectory of disease progression in the preclinical cohort. Continued research is necessary to address the complexity of cardiomyopathic progression and develop efficacious therapeutics.

Cardiomyopathies are diseases of the myocardium, often genetically determined, associated with heterogeneous phenotypes and clinical manifestations. Despite significant progress in the understanding of these conditions, available treatments mostly target late complications, whereas approaches that promise to interfere with the primary mechanisms and natural history are just beginning to surface. The past decade has witnessed the establishment of large international cardiomyopathy registries, paralleled by advances in cardiac imaging and genetic testing, deeper understanding of the pathophysiology, and growing involvement by the pharmaceutical industry. As a result, the number of molecular interventions under scrutiny is increasing sharply.

With an increasing understanding of genetic defects leading to cardiomyopathy, focus is shifting to correcting these underlying genetic defects. One approach involves treating mutant RNA through antisense oligonucleotides; the first drug has received regulatory approval to treat specific mutations associated with Duchenne muscular dystrophy. Gene editing is being evaluated in the preclinical setting. For inherited cardiomyopathies, genetic correction strategies require tight specificity for the mutant allele. Gene-editing methods are being tested to create deletions that may be useful to restore protein expression through the bypass of mutations that restore protein production. Site-specific gene editing, which is required to correct many point mutations, is a less efficient process than inducing deletions.

Exercise and sports are an integral part of daily life for millions of Americans, with 16% of the US population older than age 15 years engaged in sports or exercise activities (Bureau of Labor Statistics). The physical and psychological benefits of exercise are well recognized; however, high-profile cases of athletes dying suddenly on the field, often due to undiagnosed genetic cardiomyopathies, raise questions about the risks and benefits of exercise for those with cardiomyopathy.

Arrhythmogenic cardiomyopathy (AC) is an inherited heart muscle disease characterized by myocardial atrophy and fibrofatty replacement of the ventricular myocardium, at risk of sudden cardiac death, particularly in the young and athletes. Because there is no "gold standard" to reach the diagnosis of AC, multiple categories of diagnostic information have been combined, including imaging, electrocardiographic changes, arrhythmias, tissue characterization, and family history.

However, the routine use of contrast-enhanced cardiac magnetic resonance increasingly revealed left dominant AC, a variant that is not well addressed in the diagnostic criteria and still escapes clinical identification.

Infiltrative cardiomyopathies are characterized by abnormal accumulation or deposition of substances in cardiac tissue leading to cardiac dysfunction. These can be inherited, resulting from mutations in specific genes, which engender a diverse array of extracardiac features but overlapping cardiac phenotypes. This article provides an overview of each inherited infiltrative cardiomyopathy, describing the causative genes, the pathologic mechanisms involved, the resulting cardiac manifestations, and the therapies currently offered or being developed.

RASopathies are a heterogeneous group of genetic syndromes characterized by mutations in genes that regulate cellular processes, including proliferation, differentiation, survival, migration, and metabolism. Excluding congenital heart defects, hypertrophic cardiomyopathy is the most frequent cardiovascular defect in patients affected by RASopathies. A worse outcome (in terms of surgical risk and/or mortality) has been described in a specific subset of patients with RASopathy with early onset, severe hypertrophic cardiomyopathy presenting with heart failure. New short-term therapy with a mammalian target of rapamycin inhibitor has recently been used to prevent heart failure in these patients with a severe form of hypertrophic cardiomyopathy.

HEART FAILURE CLINICS

ISSUE OF RELATED INTEREST

Interventional Cardiology Clinics, July 2017 (Vol. 6, Issue 3)
Interventional Heart Failure
Srihari S. Naidu, *Editor*
Available at: http://www.interventional.theclinics.com/

THE CLINICS ARE AVAILABLE ONLINE!
Access your subscription at:
www.theclinics.com

Preface

On the Road from Gene to Therapy in Inherited Cardiomyopathies

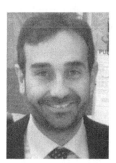
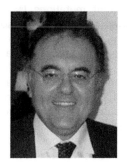
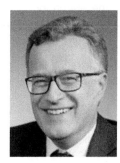
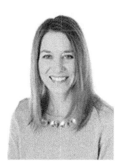

Giuseppe Limongelli, MD, PhD	Eduardo Bossone, MD, PhD, FESC, FACC	Perry M. Elliott, MBBS, MD	Sharlene M. Day, MD

Editors

The century that closed the second millennium was marked by enormous progress in all the life sciences, including medicine. In the twenty-first century, we have an unparalleled ability to observe, describe, and define clinical phenomena thanks to the discovery and progressive refinement of new tools able to determine the cause and pathophysiology of different diseases. With better recognition, many diseases previously thought to be rare have become more commonplace.

The familial nature of cardiomyopathies was first recognized in the mid-twentieth century.[1–5] One of the first families to be reported by Pare and colleagues[5] was the key to the discovery of the genetic substrate of hypertrophic cardiomyopathy when Christine and Jon Seidman applied, for the first time in cardiology, linkage techniques to discover a mutation (Arg403Glu) in MYH7 on chromosome 14.[6] This landmark paper opened the door to the era of cardiovascular genetics with a cascade of new discoveries about the cause and pathogenesis of cardiomyopathies. Today, genetic testing is an essential part of diagnosis and management of patients with cardiomyopathies, offering an invaluable tool for risk prediction, cascade genetic testing of at-risk relatives, and reproductive testing options.[7] Specialized multidisciplinary clinics, including cardiologists and genetic counselors, are now standard of care,[7] and advances in genetic testing technologies have increased the yield and accuracy of genetic testing at ever-reducing cost.[7,8]

Cardiomyopathies are a heterogeneous group of myocardial disorders in which the heart muscle is structurally and/or functionally abnormal in the absence of any condition that can explain the observed phenotype.[9] The estimated combined population prevalence of all cardiomyopathies is at least 3%.[10] Most cardiomyopathies are genetic disorders affecting the structural and functional proteins of the cardiomyocyte.[9–15] They can be primary genetic disorders of the myocardium or be part of multisystem disorders (phenocopies), such as malformation syndromes, neuromuscular disorders, mitochondrial disease, and infiltrative/storage disease.[13–15] Cardiomyopathies can be acquired, for example, following exposure to a toxin or infective agent, but even in this scenario, genetic predisposition plays an important role. The complexity of the different pathways that lead to disease means that a common classification of cardiomyopathies is still lacking, due to our inability to translate their heterogeneity and complexity into a single nosology. Nevertheless, a common language that encompasses some of the new insights on genotype and phenotype of cardiomyopathies is emerging and impacting clinical practice.

For patients, the burden of cardiomyopathies lies in the development of heart failure and sudden cardiac death. The latter is particularly relevant in children and young adults[7,16] where physical exercise can be a trigger. However, the physical and

Heart Failure Clin 14 (2018) xi–xv
https://doi.org/10.1016/j.hfc.2018.01.003
1551-7136/18/© 2018 Published by Elsevier Inc.

heartfailure.theclinics.com

psychological benefit of sport activity in daily life should be balanced case by case with the potential risk of cardiac arrest.[17,18] In the last 20 years, the use of implantable cardioverter defibrillators (ICD) has transformed primary and secondary prevention, although risk stratification for primary prevention and complications related to ICD implantation still represents challenges. Much work on risk prediction focuses on the search for new biomarkers, such as high-resolution imaging with tissue characterization. Efforts to improve the risk/benefit of ICD implantation focus on new technologies such as subcutaneous ICD leads. The role of genotype in risk stratification for sudden cardiac death is still unclear, but molecular autopsy (proband genetic testing performed on postmortem DNA) can be a valuable tool for clarification of the cause of death and for allowing appropriate screening and risk stratification of family members.[7,16]

Recent practice guidelines have highlighted the important contribution of inherited cardiomyopathies to the burden of heart failure.[19] Dilated cardiomyopathy (DCM) and advanced-stage hypertrophic cardiomyopathy (HCM) and arrhythmogenic cardiomyopathy (AC) represent important causes of heart failure with reduced ejection fraction, while restrictive cardiomyopathy (RCM) and restrictive HCM represent extremes of heart failure with preserved ejection fraction (HFPEF).[20–22] Moreover, increased recognition of infiltrative disease (ie, amyloidosis) is revealing common and potentially treatable causes of HFPEF in specific subgroups and ethnic populations.[23,24] The future development of heart failure services will lie in closer collaboration between heart failure and cardiomyopathy specialists within multidisciplinary teams. Progress will also come from large-scale collaborations, registries, and national electronic health records which it is hoped will provide the power to appreciate cumulative disease burden, define accurate risk estimates for adverse events, and determine how genotype impacts disease.[9]

The mechanism by which gene mutations lead to protein and cell dysfunction and clinical disease is an area of active investigation. Phenotypic characterization of preclinical sarcomere gene mutation carriers has yielded insights into the earliest biomechanical defects that link pathogenic variants to cardiac remodeling and dysfunction.[11,25] For example, hyperdynamic ventricular contraction and diastolic dysfunction are the earliest identified biomechanical defects in human HCM, while systolic dysfunction is the first sign of pathophysiology in DCM.[11,25] Sarcomeric protein gene mutations can result in either phenotype, but functional studies have shown that disease may relate directly to their impact on different functional domains and protein-protein interactions.[11,25] Another recent discovery is that titin truncating variants, yielding titin haploinsufficiency, represent the most common cause of familial DCM.[11,25–27] Experimental data support the hypothesis that titin is critical for sarcomere assembly and content and that mutations lead to an abnormal and inadequate stress response (for example, during increased hemodynamic load in pregnancy).[11,25–27] Considerable progress has also been made in understanding AC caused by genes encoding proteins of the cardiac desmosomes, which lead to disruption of intermyocyte connections and alteration of intracellular signal transduction. Wnt/β catenin and Hippo signaling pathways have been implicated in disease pathogenesis as well as known regulators of adipogenesis, fibrogenesis, and apoptosis, the main cellular mechanisms underpinning the disease phenotype.

Therapies in cardiomyopathies vary according to the disease stage. Some treatments are essentially palliative, but in DCM, ACE inhibitors and β-blockers delay progression and improve prognosis. Disease-modifiying treatments have not been identified for HCM or AC, but there has been a recent surge of clinical trials testing new therapies for cardiomyopathies. One such therapy being tested for HCM is mavacampten (MYK-461; Myokardia, San Francisco, CA, USA), a small-molecule allosteric myosin inhibitor that restores contractile balance in HCM hearts by decreasing adenosine triphosphatase activity of the cardiac myosin heavy chain.[28,29] A phase 2a study has recently been completed to evaluate the efficacy, safety, and tolerability of mavacamten in subjects with symptomatic HCM and left ventricular outflow tract obstruction (NCT02842242); a large phase 2/3 study is due to start in 2018. This trial is supported by data from preclinical studies showing that in an HCM mouse model, mavacampten administered in an early stage prevented disease development (left ventricular hypertrophy, myocyte disarray, and fibrosis) and downregulated both hypertrophic and profibrotic gene expression.[28,29]

Phenotype prevention or reverse remodeling is the ultimate goal of pharmacologic therapy. Different therapies have been or are being tested in HCM. Diltiazem has shown some promise in sarcomere gene mutations carriers in a small clinical trial,[30] while no benefit was apparent with N-acetylcysteine, atorvastatin, or ranolazine analogs.[29,31–34] Valsartan is currently under investigation in the VANISH trial.[35] This trial was based on encouraging findings from a preclinical trial in which inhibiting TGF-β by neutralizing antibodies or with losartan prevented phenotypic development in mice carrying a MYH7 mutation.[36] Gene-targeted therapies are also on the horizon, enabled by recent advances in gene-editing technology. In a recent study, genetic engineering using CRISPR-Cas9 technique corrected a heterozygous MYBPC3 mutation in human preimplantation embryos.[37,38] However, the applicability of this technique to clinical practice is uncertain, in light of concerns about off-target effects and the current availability of preimplantation genetic diagnosis, which allows for implantation of genetically unaffected embryos.

Other innovative breakthroughs have emerged in the field of rare multisystem diseases, such as chaperone therapy (migalastat) for Fabry disease and antisense oligonucleotides (eteplirsen) for Duchenne muscular dystrophy, both recently approved in clinical practice.[29] New developments are underway in rasopathies, where short-term therapy with mTOR inhibitors (everolimus) has recently been used to prevent disease complications in patients with a severe form of HCM[39] and in lamin A/C disease, where a p38α inhibitor is under investigation in a phase 2 study trial of lamin A/C DCM (NCT02351856).[40]

In conclusion, almost 30 years after the discovery of the first genetic mutation for HCM, the development of new pharmacologic approaches targeting cardiomyopathies and other orphan/rare cardiac disease is closer to reality. Development of targeted therapies is enabled by new insights into clinical phenotypes and molecular pathogenesis, along with the establishment of large-scale international collaboration and engagement of the pharmaceutical industry. The road toward cardiovascular precision medicine is just beginning, with inherited and rare diseases leading the way.

Giuseppe Limongelli, MD, PhD
Department of Cardiothoracic Sciences
Università della Campania "Luigi Vanvitelll"
Monaldi Hospital, AORN Colli
Centro di Ricerca Cardiovascolare
Ospedale Monaldi, AORN Colli
Via L. Bianchi
Naples 80131, Italy

UCL Institute of Cardiovascular Science
London, UK

Eduardo Bossone, MD, PhD, FESC, FACC
'Cava de' Tirreni and Amalfi Coast'
Division of Cardiology
Heart Department
University Hospital
Salerno, Italy

Perry M. Elliott, MBBS, MD
University College London
UCL Institute of Cardiovascular Science
Barts Heart Centre
St Bartholomew's Hospital
West Smithfield
London EC1A 7BE, UK

Sharlene M. Day, MD
Department of Internal Medicine
Division of Cardiovascular Medicine
Department of Molecular and Integrative
Physiology
Program for Inherited Cardiomyopathies
Cardiovascular Center Floor 3
1500 East Medical Center Drive, SPC 5856
Ann Arbor, MI 48109, USA

E-mail addresses:
giuseppe.limongelli@unicampania.it
(G. Limongelli)
ebossone@hotmail.com (E. Bossone)
perry.elliott@ucl.ac.uk (P.M. Elliott)
sday@med.umich.edu (S.M. Day)

REFERENCES

1. Evans W. Familial cardiomegaly. Br Heart J 1949; 11(1):68–82.
2. De Matteis F, Ozzano T. Familial idiopathic cardiomegaly. Minerva Med 1954;45(43):1549–55 [in Italian].
3. Hollman A, Goodwin JF, Teare D, et al. A family with obstructive cardiomyopathy (asymmetrical hypertrophy). Br Heart J 1960;22:449–56.
4. Teare D. Asymmetrical hypertrophy of the heart in young adults. Br Heart J 1958;20(1):1–8.
5. Pare JA, Fraser RG, Pirozynski WJ, et al. Hereditary cardiovascular dysplasia. A form of familial cardiomyopathy. Am J Med 1961;31:37–62.
6. Geisterfer-Lowrance AA, Kass S, Tanigawa G, et al. A molecular basis for familial hypertrophic cardiomyopathy: a beta cardiac myosin heavy chain gene missense mutation. Cell 1990;62:999–1006.
7. Ingles JJ, Bagnall RD, Semsarian C. Genetic testing for cardiomyopathies in clinical practice. Heart Fail Clin, in press.
8. D'Argenio V, Frisso G, Precone V, et al. DNA sequence capture and next-generation sequencing for the molecular diagnosis of genetic cardiomyopathies. J Mol Diagn 2014;16(1):32–44.
9. Masarone D, Kaski JP, Pacileo G, et al. Epidemiology and clinical aspects of genetic cardiomyopathies. Heart Fail Clin, in press.
10. McKenna WJ, Maron BJ, Thiene G. Classification, epidemiology, and global burden of cardiomyopathies. Circ Res 2017;121:722–30.

11. Garfinkel AC, Seidman JG, Seidman CE. Genetic pathogenesis of hypertrophic and dilated cardiomyopathy. Heart Fail Clin, in press.

12. Basso C, Corrado D, Thiene G. Diagnostic criteria, genetics, and molecular basis of ARVC. Heart Fail Clin, in press.

13. Dhandapany PS, Razzaque MA, Muthusami U, et al. RAF1 mutations in childhood-onset dilated cardiomyopathy. Nat Genet 2014;46(6):635–9.

14. Sweet ME, Mestroni L, Taylor MRG. Genetic infiltrative cardiomyopathies. Heart Fail Clin, in press.

15. Calcagni G, Digilio MC, Adorisio R, et al. Clinical presentation and natural history of hypertrophic cardiomyopathy in Rasopathies. Heart Fail Clin, in press.

16. Bagnall RD, Weintraub RG, Ingles J, et al. A prospective study of sudden cardiac death among children and young adults. N Engl J Med 2016;374(25):2441–52.

17. Atteya G, Lampert R. Controversies surrounding exercise in genetic cardiomyopathies. Heart Fail Clin, in press.

18. Saberi S, Wheeler M, Bragg-Gresham J, et al. Effect of moderate-intensity exercise training on peak oxygen consumption in patients with hypertrophic cardiomyopathy: a randomized clinical trial. JAMA 2017;317(13):1349–57.

19. Ezekowitz JA, O'Meara E, McDonald M, et al. Comprehensive update of the Canadian Cardiovascular Society Guidelines for the management of heart failure. Can J Cardiol 2017. https://doi.org/10.1016/j.cjca.2017.08.022.

20. Pinto YM, Elliott PM, Arbustini E, et al. Proposal for a revised definition of dilated cardiomyopathy, hypokinetic non-dilated cardiomyopathy, and its implications for clinical practice: a position statement of the ESC working group on myocardial and pericardial diseases. Eur Heart J 2016;37(23):1850–8.

21. Biagini E, Olivotto I, Iascone M, et al. Significance of sarcomere gene mutations analysis in the end-stage phase of hypertrophic cardiomyopathy. Am J Cardiol 2014;114(5):769–76.

22. Limongelli G, Masarone D, Frisso G, et al. Clinical and genetic characterization of patients with hypertrophic cardiomyopathy and right atrial enlargement. J Cardiovasc Med (Hagerstown) 2017;18(4):249–54.

23. González-López E, Gallego-Delgado M, Guzzo-Merello G, et al. Wild-type transthyretin amyloidosis as a cause of heart failure with preserved ejection fraction. Eur Heart J 2015;36(38):2585–94.

24. Dungu JN, Papadopoulou SA, Wykes K, et al. Afro-Caribbean heart failure in the United Kingdom: cause, outcomes, and ATTR V122I Cardiac Amyloidosis. Circ Heart Fail 2016;9(9) [pii:e003352].

25. Lynn, ML, Lehman SJ, Tardiff, J. Biophysical derangements in genetic cardiomyopathies. Heart Fail Clin, in press.

26. Hinson JT, Chopra A, Nafissi N, et al. Titin mutations in iPS cells define sarcomere insufficiency as a cause of dilated cardiomyopathy. Science 2015;349(6251):982–6.

27. Schafer S, de Marvao A, Adami E, et al. Titin-truncating variants affect heart function in disease cohorts and the general population. Nat Genet 2016;49(1):46–53.

28. Green EM, Wakimoto H, Anderson RL, et al. A small-molecule inhibitor of sarcomere contractility suppresses hypertrophic cardiomyopathy in mice. Science 2016;351(6273):617–21.

29. Maurizi N, Ammirati E, Coppini R, et al. Clinical and molecular aspects of cardiomyopathies: emerging therapies and clinical trials. Heart Fail Clin, in press.

30. Ho CY, Lakdawala NK, Cirino AL, et al. Diltiazem treatment for pre-clinical hypertrophic cardiomyopathy sarcomere mutation carriers: a pilot randomized trial to modify disease expression. JACC Heart Fail 2015;3:180–8.

31. Lombardi R, Rodriguez G, Chen SN, et al. Resolution of established cardiac hypertrophy and fibrosis and prevention of systolic dysfunction in a transgenic rabbit model of human cardiomyopathy through thiol-sensitive mechanisms. Circulation 2009;119:1398–407.

32. Senthil V, Chen SN, Tsybouleva N, et al. Prevention of cardiac hypertrophy by atorvastatin in a transgenic rabbit model of human hypertrophic cardiomyopathy. Circ Res 2005;97:285–92.

33. Nagueh SF, Lombardi R, Tan Y, et al. Atorvastatin and cardiac hypertrophy and function in hypertrophic cardiomyopathy: a pilot study. Eur J Clin Invest 2010;40:976–83.

34. Olivotto I, Camici PG, Merlini PA, et al. Efficacy of ranolazine in patients with symptomatic hypertrophic cardiomyopathy: the "Restyle-HCM" randomised, double-blind, placebo-controlled study. Circ Heart Fail 2018;11(1):e004124.

35. Ho CY, McMurray JJV, Cirino AL, et al, VANISH Trial Investigators and Executive Committee. The design of the Valsartan for Attenuating Disease Evolution in Early Sarcomeric Hypertrophic Cardiomyopathy (VANISH) trial. Am Heart J 2017;187:145–55.

36. Teekakirikul P, Eminaga S, Toka O, et al. Cardiac fibrosis in mice with hypertrophic cardiomyopathy is mediated by non-myocyte proliferation and requires TGF-β. J Clin Invest 2010;120(10):3520–9.

37. Ma H, Marti-Gutierrez N, Park SW, et al. Correction of a pathogenic gene mutation in human embryos. Nature 2017;548(7668):413–9.

38. Ohiri JC, McNally EM. Gene editing and gene-based therapeutics for cardiomyopathies. Heart Fail Clin, in press.

39. Calcagni G, Adorisio R, Martinelli S, et al. Clinical presentation and natural history of hypertrophic cardiomyopathy in RASopathies, in press.

40. Captur G, Arbustini E, Bonne G, et al. Lamin and the heart. Heart 2017. https://doi.org/10.1136/heartjnl-2017-312338.

Epidemiology and Clinical Aspects of Genetic Cardiomyopathies

Daniele Masarone, MD, PhD[a],*, Juan Pablo Kaski, MD[b,c],
Giuseppe Pacileo, MD[a], Perry M. Elliott, MBBS, MD[c],
Eduardo Bossone, MD, PhD[d], Sharlene M. Day, MD[e],
Giuseppe Limongelli, MD, PhD[a,c,f]

KEYWORDS

- Hypertrophic cardiomyopathy • Nonischemic dilated cardiomyopathy
- Arrhythmogenic right ventricular cardiomyopathy • Restrictive cardiomyopathy • Clinical registry

KEY POINTS

- Cardiomyopathies are an increasingly recognized cause of heart failure and sudden death, particularly in young patients.
- Since their original description, major advances were achieved in the phenotype knowledge, natural history, and nosography of cardiomyopathies leading to different classification systems.
- Deeper knowledge of the natural history of the disease and its phases (preclinical, overt disease, and end-stage disease) is needed.
- Large-scale clinical registries provide the opportunity to bridge knowledge gaps and improve risk prediction and management of patients with cardiomyopathies.

INTRODUCTION

Cardiomyopathies (CMPs) are myocardial disorders in which the heart muscle is structurally and functionally abnormal in the absence of abnormal conditions that can explain the observed myocardial abnormality.[1] Although considered rare diseases, the estimated combined prevalence of all CMPs is at least 3%.[2] Furthermore, their recognition is increasing because of advances in imaging techniques[3] and greater awareness in both the lay and medical communities. CMPs are typified by clinical and genetic heterogeneity and are associated with significant morbidity and mortality.[4] In this article, the authors summarize the classification, epidemiology, and phenotypic spectrum of genetic CMPs. (**Tables 1** and **2**)

CLASSIFICATION OF CARDIOMYOPATHIES

In 1957, Brigden[5] first used the term *cardiomyopathies* to describe a group of uncommon myocardial diseases not related to coronary artery diseases. Later in the 1960s, Goodwin and colleagues[6] defined CMPs as "*myocardial diseases of unknown cause*"[6] and identified 3 different entities, namely, dilated CMP (DCM), hypertrophic CMP (HCM), and restrictive CMP (RCM).

Disclosure Statement: The authors have nothing to disclose.
[a] Cardiomyopathies and Heart Failure Unit, Monaldi Hospital, Via Leonardo Bianchi, Naples 84100, Italy; [b] Department of Cardiology, Centre for Inherited Cardiovascular Diseases, Great Ormond Street Hospital, Great Ormond Street, London WC1N 3JH, UK; [c] Department of Cardiology, UCL Institute of Cardiovascular Science, Gower Street, London WC1E 6BT, UK; [d] Cardiology Division, University of Salerno, Largo Città di Ippocrate, Salerno 84131, Italy; [e] Department of Internal Medicine, Division of Cardiovascular Medicine, University of Michigan, 1500 East Medical Center Drive, Ann Arbor, MI 48109, USA; [f] Department of Cardiothoracic Sciences, Università della Campania "Luigi Vanvitelli", Via Leonardo Bianchi, Naples 84100, Italy
* Corresponding author. Cardiomyopathies and Heart Failure Unit, Monaldi Hospital, Via Leonardo Bianchi 1, Naples, Italy.
E-mail address: danielemasarone@libero.it

Heart Failure Clin 14 (2018) 119–128
https://doi.org/10.1016/j.hfc.2017.12.007

Table 1
Classification systems for cardiomyopathies

Author/Year	CMP Definition	Classification
Goodwing/1972	Myocardial diseases of unknown cause	Hypertrophic CMP Dilated CMP Restrictive CMP
WHO/ISFC/1995	Diseases of the myocardium associated with cardiac dysfunction	Hypertrophic CMP Dilated CMP Restrictive CMP Arrhythmogenic right ventricular CMP Unclassified CMP • Fibroelastosis • Noncompacted myocardium Specific CMPs • Ischemic CMP • Valvular CMP • Hypertensive CMP • Inflammatory CMP • Metabolic CMP • Associated to general system diseases (eg, sarcoidosis) • Associated to muscular dystrophies • Associated to neuromuscular diseases • Caused by toxic reaction (eg, alcoholic CMP) • Peripartal CMP
AHA/2006	A heterogeneous group of diseases of the myocardium associated with mechanical and/or electrical dysfunction that usually (but not invariably) exhibit inappropriate ventricular hypertrophy or dilatation and are due to a variety of causes that frequently are genetic	Genetic • Hypertrophic CMP • Arrhythmogenic right ventricular CMP/ dysplasia • Left ventricular noncompaction • Channelopathies Mixed • Dilated CMP • Restrictive CMP Acquired • Inflammatory CMP • Takotsubo CMP • Peripartum CMP • Tachycardia-induced CMP

ESC/2008	A myocardial disorder in which the heart muscle is structurally and functionally abnormal, in the absence of coronary artery disease, hypertension, valvular disease, and congenital heart disease sufficient to cause the observed myocardial abnormality	Hypertrophic CMP
		• Familial
		  ○ Unknown gene
		  ○ Sarcomeric protein mutation
		  ○ Glycogen storage diseases
		  ○ Lysosomal storage disease
		  ○ Disorder of fatty acid metabolism
		  ○ Carnitine deficiency
		  ○ Mitochondrial cytopathies
		  ○ Noonan syndrome
		  ○ Leopard syndrome
		  ○ Friedreich ataxia
		  ○ Amyloid (mutated TTR)
		• Nonfamilial
		  ○ Obesity
		  ○ Infants of diabetic mothers
		  ○ Athletic training
		  ○ Amyloid (AL/prealbumin, wild-type TTR)

(continued on next page)

Author/Year	CMP Definition	Classification

		Dilated CMP
		• Familial
		  ○ Unknown gene
		  ○ Sarcomeric protein
		  ○ Z-band muscle
		  ○ LIM protein
		  ○ TCAP
		  ○ Cytoskeletal genes dystrophin
		  ○ Desmin
		  ○ Metavinculin
		  ○ Sarcoglycan complex
		  ○ Epicardin
		  ○ Nuclear membrane
		  ○ Lamin A/C
		  ○ Emerin
		  ○ Intercalated disc protein
		  ○ Mitochondrial cytopathy
		• Nonfamilial
		  ○ Myocarditis
		  ○ Kawasaki disease
		  ○ Eosinophilic
		  ○ Drugs
		  ○ Pregnancy
		  ○ Endocrine
		  ○ Nutritional
		  ○ Hypophosphatemia
		  ○ Hypocalcemia
		  ○ Alcohol
		  ○ Tachycardiomyopathy
		Restrictive CMP
		• Familial
		  ○ Tropinin I
		  ○ Desmin
		  ○ HFE
		  ○ Amyloid (mutated TTR)
		• Nonfamilial
		  ○ Sarcoidosis
		  ○ Carcinoid heart disease
		  ○ Scleroderma
		  ○ Amyloid (AL/prealbumin, wild-type TTR)
		• Arrhythmogenic right ventricular CMP
		• Unclassified CMP
		  ○ Left ventricular noncompaction
		  ○ Takotsubo CMP

WHF/2013	Heart muscle disease sufficient to cause structural and functional myocardial abnormality in the absence of coronary artery disease, hypertension, valvular disease, and congenital heart disease	Descriptive genotype-phenotype nosology system (see text for details)

Abbreviations: AHA, American Heart Association; AL, Light chain; ESC, European Society of Cardiology; ISFC, International Society and Federation of Cardiology; TCAP, Titin cap gene; TTR, Transthyretin; WHF, World Heart Federation; WHO, World Health Organization.

Table 2
Prevalence of adults and pediatric cardiomyopathies

	Pediatric	Adult
Hypertrophic CMP	Not available	Prevalence 1 per 500 to 1 per 200[a]
Dilated CMP	Not available	1 per 2700 to 1 per 250[b]
Arrhythmogenic right ventricular CMP	Not available	1 per 2000–5000
Restrictive CMP	Not available	Not available

[a] Newer techniques (ie, genetic testing, cardiac MRI) have increased recognition of the hypertrophic CMP (HCM) phenotype and improved clinical diagnosis. For these reasons, the prevalence of HCM in the general population has been estimated to be closer to 1 out of every 200.

[b] The only formal study that estimated the prevalence of dilated CMP (DCM) was the Olmsted study (~1 per 2700). This prevalence was twice the prevalence of hypertrophic cardiomyopathy (HCM), which was estimated at 19.7 per 100,000 (~1 per 5000) from the same cohort during this study period. Subsequently, multiple well-designed epidemiologic studies have shown an HCM prevalence of approximately 1 per 500. It is highly likely that the Olmsted County study also significantly underestimated the prevalence of DCM, so the estimated prevalence generated from the HCM/DCM incidence data is now considered approximately 1 per 500.

In 1996, the World Health Organization and the International Society and Federation of Cardiology[7] redefined CMPs as "*diseases of the myocardium associated with cardiac dysfunction.*" A new entity, arrhythmogenic right ventricular CMP (ARVC), was added to the classification, whereas several unclassified CMPs were highlighted, including left ventricular noncompaction (LVNC).

In the new millennium, the classification of CMPs was revisited once more by the American Heart Association (AHA) and the European Society of Cardiology (ESC) in independent initiatives. In 2006, the AHA published a scientific statement in which CMPs were defined as "*a heterogeneous group of diseases of the myocardium associated with mechanical and/or electrical dysfunction that usually (but not invariably) exhibit inappropriate ventricular hypertrophy or dilatation and are due to a variety of causes that frequently are genetic.*"[8] The writing committee maintained a distinction between primary CMPs (when disease is solely or predominantly of the heart muscle) and secondary CMPs (when myocardial involvement is associated with a multisystem disorder). In addition, primary CMPs were classified as genetic (HCM, ARVC, LVNC), acquired (peripartum, tachycardia induced, myocarditis, Takotsubo), or mixed (DCM, RCM); ion channel diseases were included as functional (ie, electrophysiologic) disorders of the cardiomyocyte.

In contrast, an ESC position statement in 2008 created a categorization system in which CMPs were still defined as "*myocardial disorders in which the heart muscle is structurally and functionally abnormal in the absence of coronary artery disease, hypertension, valvular or congenital heart disease sufficient to cause the observed myocardial abnormality.*"[9] Ion channel diseases were specifically excluded because of their lack of a structural cardiac phenotype.

The aim of the ESC document was to deliberately emphasize the distinction between genetic and nongenetic forms of disease to increase awareness of the spectrum of disorders that result in heart muscle dysfunction. Because the diagnosis of CMPs is based on a clinical phenotype, the 4 classic morphologic subgroups of hypertrophic, dilated, restrictive, and arrhythmogenic CMPs were maintained and a fifth subgroup of unclassified CMPs (including LVNC) was added. Each category was subdivided into familial and nonfamilial subsets.

The most recent classification of CMPs is that proposed by the World Heart Federation in 2013, known as the MOGE(S) classification.[10] In keeping with the ESC position statement, CMPs are defined by the presence of "*heart muscle disease sufficient to cause structural and functional myocardial abnormality in the absence of coronary artery disease, hypertension, valvular disease, and congenital heart disease.*"[9] In contrast, however, the MOGE(S) scheme includes both genotype and phenotype in the classification of CMPs.

The MOGE(S) nomenclature system has 5 attributes:

- M: Morpho-functional characteristic
- O: Organ involvement
- G: Genetic or familial inheritance pattern
- E: Etiologic annotation
- S: Functional status using stages A to D of the ACC/AHA staging and classes I to IV using the New York Heart Association (NYHA) functional classification (The descriptor S is optional but may come in handy for the description of early CMP.)
- MD stands for dilated CMP, MH for HCM, MA for ARVC, MR for RCM, and MLNVC for LVNC.
- OH stands for heart only, OH + M for heart and skeletal muscle, OH + A for heart and nervous system, and so on.
- GAD stands for autosomal dominant, GAR for autosomal recessive, GXL for X-linked, and so on.

- EG stands for genetic cause with subgroups like EG-MYH7[p. Arg403Glu] for one variety of HCM.
- S^{B-I} stands for a variety of CMPs in heart failure stage B and functional class I and so on.

For example, M$_H$ O$_H$ G$_{AD}$ E$_{G-MYH7[p. Arg403Glu]}$ S$_{B-I}$ represents morpho-functional phenotype (M): HCM (H); organ (O) involvement: heart (H); genetic/familial (G) with autosomal dominant (AD) transmission; cause (E): genetic (G) and caused by the p.Arg403Glu mutation of the MYH7 gene, ACC/AHA stage (S) B, NYHA I.

EPIDEMIOLOGY OF CARDIOMYOPATHIES

It is now clear that most of the CMPs are relatively common in everyday clinical practice. HCM is probably the most common subtype with a prevalence of 1 per 500 to 1 per 200[11,12] in adults of all races. Disease expression usually occurs in adolescents and young adults, whereas it is thought to be less common in young children, in whom other causes, such as metabolic storage diseases, need to be considered.[13] The historical estimated prevalence of DCM is 1 per 2500; however, more recent estimates suggest a substantially higher prevalence of approximately 1 or more in 250 individuals.[14] In children, DCM is less common, with an overall annual incidence of 0.57 cases per 100,000 person-years.[15] In the pediatric age group, the incidence of DCM is greater in the first year of life (4.58 per 100,000) than during childhood and adolescence (0.34 per 100,000); the prevalent causes are myocarditis,

neuromuscular disorders, and inborn errors of metabolism.[16]

The prevalence of ARVC has not been systematically studied but is estimated at 1 per 2000 to 5000 in adults,[17] whereas in childhood ARVC is rare and disease expression usually occurs during adolescence and early adulthood.

Finally, RCM represents a very small fraction (less than 5%) of all CMPs in Western countries, both in pediatric[18] and in adult populations, although they are more common in certain regions, for example, endomyocardial fibrosis is a relatively common cause of heart failure in equatorial Africa.

CLINICAL ASPECTS OF CARDIOMYOPATHIES

CMPs represent a frequent cause of heart failure and sudden death, particularly in children and young adults (**Fig. 1**). In this section, the authors briefly summarize the clinical phenotype of CMPs.

Hypertrophic Cardiomyopathy

The diagnosis of HCM is based on the demonstration of unexplained myocardial hypertrophy, which in practice means a left ventricular (LV) wall thickness of 1.5 cm or greater in an adult of normal size; but less stringent criteria are applied to first-degree relatives of an unequivocally affected individual.[19] Most patients have familial disease, usually with AD inheritance. Mutations in genes encoding proteins of the cardiac sarcomere are the most common cause (~60% of all cases, >90% of genetically defined cases).[20] Symptomatic presentation occurs at any age, with

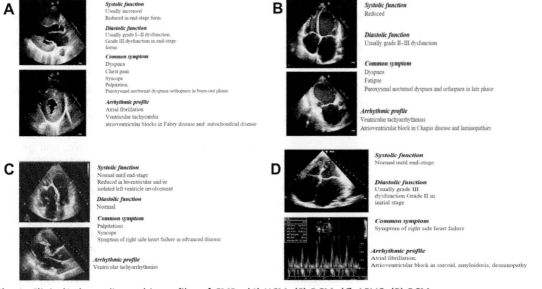

Fig. 1. Clinical/echocardiographic profiles of CMPs. (*A*) HCM. (*B*) DCM. (*C*) ARVC. (*D*) RCM.

breathlessness on exertion, chest pain, palpitation, syncope, or sudden death.[21] In children and adolescents, the diagnosis is often made during screening of siblings and offspring of affected family members. The 12-lead electrocardiography (ECG) is a sensitive but nonspecific diagnostic test. Echocardiography reveals LV hypertrophy that is symmetric or asymmetric and localized most commonly to both the septum and free wall with relative sparing of the posterior wall.[22] β-adrenoceptor blockers and non dihydropyridine calcium antagonists are the main symptomatic pharmacologic therapies, particularly for patients with LV outflow tract obstruction.[23] Surgical myectomy via a transaortic approach is considered for patients with symptomatic LV outflow-tract obstruction that is refractory to medical therapy.[24] Injection of alcohol into the septal artery that supplies the septal muscle is an alternative percutaneous technique that can be used in patients with suitable cardiac and coronary anatomy.[25] The overall annual cardiovascular mortality is 1% to 2% per year, with sudden cardiac death (SCD) (1%), heart failure (0.5%), and thromboembolism (0.1%) the main causes.[26,27] Prevention of sudden death relies on risk factor stratification to identify high-risk individuals and targeted therapy with implantable cardioverter defibrillators (ICD).[28] Atrial fibrillation is very common in patients with HCM, affecting approximately 20% to 25% of the population.[29]

Dilated Cardiomyopathy

DCM is defined by dilatation and impaired systolic function of the left or both ventricles not attributable to coronary artery disease, valvular abnormalities, or pericardial disease.[30] Up to 50% of cases are familial, with many disease-causing gene mutations described.[31]

The diagnosis relies on demonstration of an increase in LV end-diastolic dimensions greater than 2 standard deviations greater than the mean and an ejection fraction less than 50%.[32]

The initial presentation is usually with symptoms of cardiac failure, but some individuals may present for the first time with arrhythmia and/or systemic thromboembolism.

Symptomatic therapy is with diuretics, mineralocorticoid receptor antagonists, angiotensin-converting enzyme inhibitors, and β-blockers.[33] Anticoagulation with warfarin is advised in patients in whom an intracardiac thrombus is identified or those with a history of thromboembolism. ICDs are warranted if sustained or symptomatic ventricular arrhythmias are documented and for primary prophylaxis in selected high-risk patients.[34] Cardiac resynchronization therapy can improve symptoms

and the prognosis in selected patients with broad QRS duration,[35] and cardiac transplantation may be necessary for adults and pediatric patients with progressive deterioration.[36,37]

Restrictive Cardiomyopathy

RCMs are defined by restrictive ventricular physiology in the presence of normal or reduced diastolic volumes of one or both ventricles, normal or reduced systolic volumes, and normal ventricular wall thickness.[38] In developed countries amyloidosis is the most common cause, whereas in the tropics it is endomyocardial fibrosis. Familial RCM is usually caused by sarcomere protein gene mutations.[39]

The presentation is usually insidious with symptoms of pulmonary congestion and/or mitral regurgitation, hepatomegaly, ascites, and tricuspid regurgitation.[40] Atrial fibrillation is common. Echocardiography typically shows that ventricular dimensions and wall thickness are normal but the atria are grossly enlarged. Congestive symptoms from increased right atrial pressure can be improved with diuretics, but the prognosis of advanced disease is poor.[41]

Arrhythmogenic Cardiomyopathy

Arrhythmogenic cardiomyopathy (AC) is a heart muscle disease characterized by progressive fibrofatty replacement of right ventricular (RV) and LV myocardium associated with ventricular arrhythmia, heart failure, and SCD.[42] Because the originally described disease phenotype was characterized by predominant RV involvement, this disease was first named ARVC. The current term, AC, encompasses not only right predominant but also left predominant and biventricular involvement that have been increasingly recognized variants over the last several years.[43] AC is caused by mutations in desmosomal genes in at least 50% of cases.[44] The symptomatic presentation is usually with palpitations or syncope from sustained ventricular arrhythmia, but the first presentation of the disease may be with SCD. There is no single diagnostic test; the diagnosis is based on the presence of criteria encompassing structural, histologic, electrocardiographic, arrhythmic, and genetic parameters.[45–47] Risk stratification for SCD is critical for the management of patients with AC, but it is challenging to identify those who should have an ICD implanted. Patients with aborted SCD, sustained ventricular tachycardia (VT), or severe RV or LV dysfunction are high risk and warrant implantation of an ICD. Syncope, nonsustained VT, and moderate ventricular dysfunction are major risk factors for which an ICD should be strongly considered. Those with minor risk factors (abnormal ECG, male sex, proband status, positive electrophysiology study, complex genotype) may also warrant consideration of an ICD. Healthy gene carriers without any risk factors are low risk and should have an ICD implanted.[48]

REGISTRIES ON CARDIOMYOPATHIES

Until recently, most information about the presentation and natural history of individual disorders came from cohort studies in a small number of single centers in Europe and the United States. In order to derive data from less selected cohorts and expand the diversity and scope of the effort, new initiatives based on large longitudinal disease registries and national electronic health records are being conducted in several countries. Large-scale collaboration and comprehensive prospective data gathering provide the power needed to appreciate cumulative disease burden, define accurate risk estimates for adverse events, and determine how genotype impacts disease. Here, the authors highlight a few of the multicenter, international ongoing efforts on this front.

Pediatric Cardiomyopathy Registry

In 1994, the Pediatric Cardiomyopathy Registry (PCMR; https://clinicaltrials.gov/ct2/show/NCT00005391), a large, multicenter, observational study of primary and idiopathic CMPs in children, was funded by the National Heart, Lung, and Blood Institute to study the epidemiology and clinical presentation of pediatric CMPs (<18 years old). The registry has evolved, adding a retrospective cohort of children, with the aim to describe the clinical course and predictors of outcomes. Expanding the potential goals, a collaboration with the Pediatric Heart Transplant Study Group was formed to examine the effect of cardiac transplantation on the clinical course of CMP. The collection of blood and cardiac tissue specimens was added to investigate the relationship of a genetic and viral disease background to clinical outcomes.[49] Currently, data from more than 3500 pediatric patients have been collected.[50] PCMR has provided insight into the incidence of, and risk factors for, pediatric CMP, the prevalence of heart failure at diagnosis, survival and transplant outcomes, and determinants of functional status.[50]

EURObservational Research Programme–European Society of Cardiology

In 2009, the ESC launched the EURObservational Research Programme (EORP; https://www.escardio.org/Research/Registries-&-surveys/Observational-registry-programme) with the aim of improving the understanding of medical practice by collecting observational data using robust methodologic procedures. The EORP CMP registry is a prospective, multicenter, observational study of patients presenting to referral CMP centers in European countries. Consistent with published data, HCM is the most frequently recorded CMP in the registry, followed by DCM, ARVC, and RCM. Although rare, LVNC was most commonly reported in patients with DCM. In the 3 most common CMP subtypes, most patients were diagnosed before 50 years of age, a trend that was most evident for ARVC. The age trend was reversed in patients with RCM, reflecting the high proportion of patients in this group with amyloidosis. There was a skew toward an earlier diagnosis in men for HCM, DCM, and ARVC and in women for RCM.

A major finding in EORP is the large proportion of patients in whom familial disease is reported. This finding is particularly striking given that only 15% of patients were diagnosed as the result of family screening, illustrating the delay in referring individuals with a family history for further evaluation. A large proportion of patients in the registry underwent genetic testing with a high diagnostic yield showing that, at least within specialist CMP centers, genetic evaluation is an established part of routine practice.[51]

More than a quarter of all patients in the EORP had an ICD at enrollment, but the proportion in ARVC was 60% (predominantly for primary prophylaxis). This high rate of ICD implantation might reflect a bias toward patients with more severe disease in the registry but may also reflect the lack of clear guidelines on ICD implantation in this disease.

The EORP registry has now been extended to include pediatric patients and individuals with clinically suspected myocarditis.

Sarcomeric Human Cardiomyopathy Registry

The Sarcomeric Human Cardiomyopathy Registry (SHaRe; https://theshareregistry.org/) is the first example of a multicenter international registry aiming to create a translational, personalized approach, from basic to clinic, on the specific theme of sarcomeric CMPs. Highly curated data sets from experienced centers were harmonized to create a comprehensive, collaborative registry, currently including greater than 12,000 patients and family members and spanning greater than 24,000 patient-years. Prospective longitudinal clinical and genetic data on probands and families with HCM and DCM are collected.[52] SHaRe is funded by research grants from MyoKardia, Inc (http://www.myokardia.com/), bringing together the world's leading cardiologists and geneticists from the United States, Europe, and South America.

SHaRe has provided insight into the considerable cumulative burden of adverse outcomes in HCM, largely dominated by heart failure and atrial fibrillation (Day Sharlene, unpublished data, 2018). However, complications are typically delayed for one or more decades following diagnosis. Younger age at diagnosis and the presence of a pathogenic sarcomere gene mutation were identified as powerful multivariate predictors of adverse outcomes, including heart failure, atrial fibrillation, and ventricular arrhythmias. Even patients with sarcomere variants of uncertain significance (~9% of genotype cohort) were found to have an increased risk of adverse outcomes compared with those patients without identified variants (genotype negative), highlighting the importance of genotyping in clinical risk prediction. Future analyses of the SHaRe cohort will focus on specific clinical and genetic HCM subpopulations, refining risk prediction for adverse outcomes, and expanding to the DCM cohort.

Other CMP registries include the Hypertrophic Cardiomyopathy Registry,[53] which will incorporate a core-protocol cardiac MRI in addition to standard clinical factors for risk prediction in HCM; a Canadian national ARVC registry (NCT01804699); a European ARVC registry[54]; an ARVC patient registry at Johns Hopkins[55]; and an ARVC registry at the Mayo Clinic and Cambridge University (NCT03049254).

SUMMARY

CMPs represent a fascinating but complex area in the wide panorama of heart disorders.

Recent advances have led to an understanding of the natural history and to some effective therapies for CMPs; however, a deeper knowledge of the natural history of the disease and its phases (preclinical, overt disease, and end-stage disease) is needed. Clinical registries provide the opportunity to bridge knowledge gaps and improve risk prediction and management of patients with CMPs and their family members in the future.

REFERENCES

1. Braunwald E. Cardiomyopathies an overview. Circ Res 2017;121:711–21.

2. McKenna WJ, Maron BJ, Thiene G. Classification, epidemiology, and global burden of cardiomyopathies. Circ Res 2017;121:722–30.

3. Jan MF, Tajik AJ. Modern imaging techniques in cardiomyopathies. Circ Res 2017;121:874–91.

4. Ezekowitz JA, O'Meara E, McDonald MA, et al. 2017 comprehensive update of the Canadian cardiovascular society guidelines for the management of heart failure. Can J Cardiol 2017;33: 1342–433.

5. Brigden W. Uncommon myocardial diseases: the non-coronary cardiomyopathies. Lancet 1957;273: 1179–84, 1243–9.

6. Goodwin JF, Gordon H, Hollman A, et al. Clinical aspects of cardiomyopathy. Br Med J 1961;1:69–79.

7. Richardson P, McKenna W, Bristow M, et al. Report of the 1995 World Health Organization/International Society and Federation of Cardiology task force on the definition and classification of cardiomyopathies. Circulation 1996;93:841–2.

8. Maron BJ, Towbin JA, Thiene G, et al. American Heart Association; Council on Clinical Cardiology, Heart Failure and Transplantation Committee; Quality of Care and Outcomes Research and Functional Genomics and Translational Biology Interdisciplinary Working Groups; Council on Epidemiology and Prevention. Contemporary definitions and classification of the cardiomyopathies: an American Heart Association scientific statement from the council on clinical cardiology, heart failure and transplantation committee; quality of care and outcomes research and functional genomics and translational biology interdisciplinary working groups; and council on epidemiology and prevention. Circulation 2006;113: 1807–16.

9. Elliott P, Andersson B, Arbustini E, et al. Classification of the cardiomyopathies: a position statement from the European Society of Cardiology working group on myocardial and pericardial diseases. Eur Heart J 2008;29:270–6.

10. Arbustini E, Narula N, Dec GW, et al. The MOGE(S) classification for a phenotype-genotype nomenclature of cardiomyopathy: endorsed by the World Heart Federation. J Am Coll Cardiol 2013;62: 2046–72.

11. Maron BJ, Gardin JM, Flack JM, et al. Prevalence of hypertrophic cardiomyopathy in a general population of young adults. Echocardiographic analysis of 4111 subjects in the CARDIA Study. Coronary artery risk development in (young) adults. Circulation 1995;92(4):785–9.

12. Frisso G, Limongelli G, Pacileo G, et al. A child cohort study from southern Italy enlarges the genetic spectrum of hypertrophic cardiomyopathy. Clin Genet 2009;76:91–101.

13. Colan SD. Hypertrophic cardiomyopathy in childhood. Heart Fail Clin 2010;6:433–44.

14. Bozkurt B, Colvin M, Cook J, et al. American Heart Association Committee on Heart Failure and Transplantation of the Council on Clinical Cardiology; Council on Cardiovascular Disease in the Young; Council on Cardiovascular and Stroke Nursing;

Council on Epidemiology and Prevention; and Council on Quality of Care and Outcomes Research. Current diagnostic and treatment strategies for specific dilated cardiomyopathies: a scientific statement from the American Heart Association. Circulation 2016;134:579–646.

15. Masarone D, Valente F, Rubino M, et al. Pediatric heart failure: a practical guide to diagnosis and management. Pediatr Neonatol 2017;58:303–12.

16. Hsu DT, Canter CE. Dilated cardiomyopathy and heart failure in children. Heart Fail Clin 2010;6: 415–32.

17. Marcus FI, McKenna WJ, Sherrill D, et al. Diagnosis of arrhythmogenic right ventricular cardiomyopathy/ dysplasia: proposed modification of the task force criteria. Circulation 2010;121:1533–41.

18. Lee TM, Hsu DT, Kantor P, et al. Pediatric cardiomyopathies. Circ Res 2017;121:855–73.

19. Sen-Chowdhry S, Jacoby D, Moon JC, et al. Update on hypertrophic cardiomyopathy and a guide to the guidelines. Nat Rev Cardiol 2016; 13:651–75.

20. Sabater-Molina M, Pérez-Sánchez I, Hernández Del Rincón JP, et al. Genetics of hypertrophic cardiomyopathy: a review of current state. Clin Genet 2018; 93(1):3–14.

21. Marian AJ, Braunwald E. Hypertrophic cardiomyopathy: genetics, pathogenesis, clinical manifestations, diagnosis, and therapy. Circ Res 2017;121: 749–70.

22. Losi MA, Nistri S, Galderisi M, et al. Echocardiography in patients with hypertrophic cardiomyopathy: usefulness of old and new techniques in the diagnosis and pathophysiological assessment. Cardiovasc Ultrasound 2010;8:77–85.

23. Naghi JJ, Siegel RJ. Medical management of hypertrophic cardiomyopathy. Rev Cardiovasc Med 2010; 11:202–17.

24. Hang D, Nguyen A, Schaff HV. Surgical treatment for hypertrophic cardiomyopathy: a historical perspective. Ann Cardiothorac Surg 2017;6:318–28.

25. Spirito P, Rossi J, Maron BJ. Alcohol septal ablation: in which patients and why? Ann Cardiothorac Surg 2017;6:369–75.

26. Spirito P, Chiarella F, Carratino L, et al. Clinical course and prognosis of hypertrophic cardiomyopathy in an outpatient population. N Engl J Med 1989; 320:749–53.

27. Maron MS, Rowin EJ, Olivotto I, et al. Contemporary natural history and management of nonobstructive hypertrophic cardiomyopathy. J Am Coll Cardiol 2016;67:1399–405.

28. Trivedi A, Knight BP. ICD therapy for primary prevention in hypertrophic cardiomyopathy. Arrhythm Electrophysiol Rev 2016;5:188–96.

29. Guttman OP, Rahman MS, O'Mahony C, et al. Atrial fibrillation and thromboembolism in patients with hypertrophic cardiomyopathy: systematic review. Heart 2014;100(6):465–72.

30. Mathew T, Williams L, Navaratnam G, et al. Diagnosis and assessment of dilated cardiomyopathy: a guideline protocol from the British Society of Echocardiography. Echo Res Pract 2017;4:1–13.

31. Hershberger RE, Morales A, Siegfried JD. Clinical and genetic issues in dilated cardiomyopathy: a review for genetics professionals. Genet Med 2010;12: 655–67.

32. Elliott P. Diagnosis and management of dilated cardiomyopathy. Heart 2000;84:106–12.

33. Ponikowski P, Voors AA, Anker SD, et al. 2016 ESC guidelines for the diagnosis and treatment of acute and chronic heart failure: the task force for the diagnosis and treatment of acute and chronic heart failure of the European Society of Cardiology (ESC). Developed with the special contribution of the Heart Failure Association (HFA) of the ESC. Eur J Heart Fail 2016;18:891–975.

34. González-Torrecilla E, Arenal A, Atienza F, et al. Current Indications for implantable cardioverter defibrillators in non-ischemic cardiomyopathies and channelopathies. Rev Recent Clin Trials 2015;10(2):111–27.

35. Masarone D, Limongelli G, Ammendola E, et al. Cardiac resynchronization therapy in cardiomyopathies. J Cardiovasc Med (Hagerstown) 2014;15:92–9.

36. Cheng A, Slaughter MS. Heart transplantation. J Thorac Dis 2014;6:1105–9.

37. Schweiger M, Stiasny B, Dave H, et al. Pediatric heart transplantation. J Thorac Dis 2015;7:552–9.

38. Muchtar E, Blauwet LA, Gertz MA. Restrictive cardiomyopathy: genetics, pathogenesis, clinical manifestations, diagnosis, and therapy. Circ Res 2017; 121:819–37.

39. Sen-Chowdhry S, Syrris P, McKenna WJ. Genetics of restrictive cardiomyopathy. Heart Fail Clin 2010;6: 179–86.

40. Nihoyannopoulos P, Dawson D. Restrictive cardiomyopathies. Eur J Echocardiogr 2009;10:23–33.

41. Kushwaha SS, Fallon JT, Fuster V. Restrictive cardiomyopathy. N Engl J Med 1997;336:267–76.

42. Corrado D, Link MS, Calkins H. Arrhythmogenic right ventricular cardiomyopathy. N Engl J Med 2017;376:61–72.

43. Corrado D, Basso C, Judge DP. Arrhythmogenic cardiomyopathy. Circ Res 2017;121:784–802.

44. Marcus FI, Edson S, Towbin JA. Genetics of arrhythmogenic right ventricular cardiomyopathy: a practical guide for physicians. J Am Coll Cardiol 2013; 61:1945–8.

45. Limongelli G, Rea A, Masarone D, et al. Right ventricular cardiomyopathies: a multidisciplinary approach to diagnosis. Echocardiography 2015; 32:75–94.

46. Corrado D, Wichter T, Link MS, et al. Treatment of arrhythmogenic right ventricular cardiomyopathy/

dysplasia: an international task force consensus statement. Circulation 2015;132:441–53.

47. Zorzi A, Rigato I, Bauce B, et al. Arrhythmogenic right ventricular cardiomyopathy: risk stratification and indications for defibrillator therapy. Curr Cardiol Rep 2016;18:57–63.

48. Calkins H, Corrado D, Marcus F. Risk stratification in arrhythmogenic right ventricular cardiomyopathy. Circulation 2017;136:2068–82.

49. Wilkinson JD, Sleeper LA, Alvarez JA, et al. The pediatric cardiomyopathy registry: 1995-2007. Prog Pediatr Cardiol 2008;25:31–6.

50. Wilkinson JD, Landy DC, Colan SD, et al. The pediatric cardiomyopathy registry and heart failure: key results from the first 15 years. Heart Fail Clin 2010; 6:401–13.

51. Elliott P, Charron P, Blanes JR, et al. European cardiomyopathy pilot registry: EURObservational Research Programme of the European Society of Cardiology. Eur Heart J 2016;37:164–73.

52. Furqan A, Arscott P, Girolami F, et al. Care in specialized centers and data sharing increase agreement in hypertrophic cardiomyopathy genetic test interpretation. Circ Cardiovasc Genet 2017;10: 158–70.

53. Kramer CM, Appelbaum E, Desai MY. Hypertrophic cardiomyopathy registry: the rationale and design of an international, observational study of hypertrophic cardiomyopathy. Am Heart J 2015;170:223–30.

54. Basso C, Wichter T, Danieli GA, et al. Arrhythmogenic right ventricular cardiomyopathy: clinical registry and database, evaluation of therapies, pathology registry, DNA banking. Eur Heart J 2004; 25:531–4.

55. Groeneweg JA, Bhonsale A, James CA, et al. Clinical Presentation, Long-Term Follow-Up, and Outcomes of 1001 Arrhythmogenic Right Ventricular Dysplasia/Cardiomyopathy Patients and Family Members. Circ Cardiovasc Genet. 2015; 8:437–46.

Genetic Testing for Cardiomyopathies in Clinical Practice

Jodie Ingles, PhD, MPH[a,b,c],*, Richard D. Bagnall, PhD[a,b],
Christopher Semsarian, MBBS, PhD, MPH[a,b,c]

KEYWORDS

- Hypertrophic cardiomyopathy • Dilated cardiomyopathy
- Arrhythmogenic right ventricular cardiomyopathy • Genetic testing • Genetic counseling

KEY POINTS

- Genetic testing is a valuable part of management of families with inherited cardiomyopathies.
- Interpretation of variants is a key challenge, although efforts are being made to ensure a standardized approach.
- Public sharing of variant data is necessary to allow us to gain the greatest value of cardiac genetic testing.
- Care should be taken at all points in the genetic testing process to minimize potential harms.
- A specialized multidisciplinary clinic incorporating cardiologists and genetic counselors at minimum is the ideal model of care for families with inherited cardiomyopathies.

Genetic testing for inherited cardiomyopathies plays an increasingly valuable role in family management. As understanding of the genetic architecture of these diseases continues to grow, so does the ability to use genetics in the clinical setting. At present, many genetic testing options exist, ranging from targeted panels to more comprehensive approaches, such as exome and genome sequencing. Advances in sequencing technology have allowed faster and more affordable gene tests, and this has translated to greater uptake worldwide. With the challenges of interpreting the numerous variants that are identified through comprehensive testing methods well described,[1–3] collective international efforts to ensure a standardized approach are beginning to be realized. The ultimate benefit of this will be greater certainty around the genetic causes of inherited cardiomyopathies, translating to better care of patients and their families.

This article aims to provide an overview of the current state of genetic testing for inherited cardiomyopathies, highlighting the considerable benefit for patients and their families when used with care and in a center with specialized multidisciplinary expertise as well as discussing the challenges and the collective efforts aimed at overcoming these.

J. Ingles is a recipient of a Heart Foundation of Australia Future Leader Fellowship (#100833). C. Semsarian is the recipient of a National Health and Medical Research Council (NHMRC) Practitioner Fellowship (#1059156). Disclosure: The authors have nothing to disclose.
^a Agnes Ginges Centre for Molecular Cardiology, Centenary Institute, Sydney, New South Wales, Australia; ^b Sydney Medical School, University of Sydney, Sydney, New South Wales, Australia; ^c Department of Cardiology, Royal Prince Alfred Hospital, Sydney, New South Wales, Australia
* Corresponding author. Agnes Ginges Centre for Molecular Cardiology, Centenary Institute, Locked Bag 6, Newtown, New South Wales 2042, Australia.
E-mail address: j.ingles@centenary.org.au

Heart Failure Clin 14 (2018) 129–137
https://doi.org/10.1016/j.hfc.2017.12.001

GENETIC BASIS OF INHERITED CARDIOMYOPATHIES AND ROLE OF GENETIC TESTING

Inherited cardiomyopathies are clinically and genetically heterogeneous diseases with a combined prevalence of at least 1 in 200 to 500 in the general population.[4–7] Genetic testing does not identify an underlying cause of disease in all families, with the diagnostic yield ranging from 20% to 50% (**Table 1**). Some gene-elusive cases may be solved by discovery of new genes in the future; however, there is growing recognition that many are likely to represent nonfamilial disease subtypes.[8–10]

Hypertrophic cardiomyopathy (HCM) is the most prevalent of the inherited cardiomyopathies and recognized as a disease of the sarcomere.[7,11] Genetic testing typically involves a minimum of 8 sarcomere and additional phenocopy genes, although approximately 80% who test positive have causative variants in *MYBPC3* and *MYH7*.[12,13] The diagnostic yield when testing the index case (proband) with a definite clinical diagnosis of HCM is approximately 30% to 40%, although depending on several factors, such as positive family history and age at diagnosis.[8,14]

Familial dilated cardiomyopathy (DCM) is due to numerous underlying disease mechanisms[7] and in contrast to HCM the underlying genetics can be more difficult to elucidate. Causative genes have historically included a long list of candidates; however, newer sequencing approaches have allowed this to be narrowed considerably.[15,16] At present, truncating variants in *TTN* (*TTNtv*) have been shown to account for 20% to 25% of familial DCM, the largest proportion of cases with a genetic diagnosis.[17] Variants in *LMNA* account for 5% to 10% of familial DCM and often present clinically with conduction disease.[18]

Arrhythmogenic right ventricular cardiomyopathy (ARVC) is characterized by progressive fibrofatty replacement of the myocardium, affecting the right and sometimes left ventricles.[19] Genetically, it is caused by variants in desmosome genes. To date, 6 genes are known to cause ARVC, although variants in *PKP2* account for the largest proportion of cases.[20] Loss-of-function variants in *DSP* are also an important cause and more likely to result in left-sided ARVC and/or DCM.[21]

Inherited cardiomyopathies are typically inherited as an autosomal dominant trait. Clinical heterogeneity is a hallmark feature, with some patients presenting with minimal or no symptoms, whereas others develop severe heart failure requiring cardiac transplantation or sudden cardiac death. Sudden cardiac death can occur as one of the first presentations of disease. Among postmortem series, inherited heart diseases contribute to a majority of causes of sudden cardiac death among those aged less than 35 years.[22] Approximately 40% of cases remain unexplained even after comprehensive postmortem investigation, termed sudden unexplained death, and are presumed to be an inherited primary arrhythmogenic disorder. A further 16% are due to inherited cardiomyopathies.

THE PROCESS OF CARDIAC GENETIC TESTING

Cardiac genetic testing is performed in 2 stages. The first, proband genetic testing, involves identifying the individual in a family with the most overt clinical phenotype. The proband's DNA sample undergoes sequencing of several cardiac genes to elucidate the underlying genetic cause. If a causative variant is identified, this can then be used as a valuable tool in the family, allowing the second stage, known as cascade genetic testing. Genetic testing yields for inherited cardiomyopathies are shown in (**Fig. 1**).

Proband Genetic Testing

A blood sample is collected from the proband after pretest genetic counseling and informed consent, which is then sent to a clinical testing laboratory. Several genes are sequenced to try to identify a rare sequence change that can be attributed as the cause of disease. The size of the gene panel tested varies, with a current trend to include more genes. This means genetic testing is often comprehensive, although comprising many genes with little or no disease association. The turnaround time for a result may be approximately 8 weeks to 12 weeks. Generating the genetic report can be challenging, requiring clinical interpretation of the variants and their potential impact on clinical

---

Table 1
Genetic basis of inherited cardiomyopathies

Phenotype	Genes	Diagnostic Yield of Genetic Testing
HCM	*MYBPC3, MYH7, TNNT2, TNNI3, TPM1, MYL2, MYL3, ACTC1*	30%–50%
Familial DCM	*TTN, LMNA, PLN*	20%–30%
ARVC	*PKP2, DSP, DSC2, DSG2, JUP, TMEM43*	50%

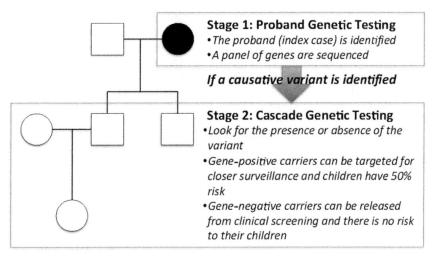

Stage 1: Proband Genetic Testing
• *The proband (index case) is identified*
• *A panel of genes are sequenced*

If a causative variant is identified

Stage 2: Cascade Genetic Testing
• *Look for the presence or absence of the variant*
• *Gene-positive carriers can be targeted for closer surveillance and children have 50% risk*
• *Gene-negative carriers can be released from clinical screening and there is no risk to their children*

Fig. 1. Stages of cardiac genetic testing.

disease. From a clinical perspective, there are 3 possible outcomes to consider: (1) a causative variant is identified, (2) a variant of uncertain significance is found, or (3) no variants of interest are identified, also known as an indeterminate result.

Cascade Genetic Testing

The clearest benefit of cardiac genetic testing is for clarifying risk to asymptomatic family members.[6] If a causative variant is identified in the proband, then this can be used as a tool to test for the presence or absence of the variant in a family. This is performed in a stepwise fashion, beginning with those relatives most closely related (ie, first-degree relatives, such as parents, siblings, or children of a proband). Those who test positive can be targeted for closer clinical surveillance, although there is growing awareness many will remain nonpenetrant gene carriers. Importantly, the increased risk to their relatives can be clarified, allowing more directed clinical screening and further cascade genetic testing options. Those who test negative can be released from all future clinical surveillance and reassured they are not at risk. Likewise, their children are not at risk of disease. The ability to inform relatives they are gene negative cannot be underestimated. Not only does it alleviate unnecessary worry but also it potentially saves years of health care costs associated with clinical surveillance. This is a driving factor behind health economic analyses in HCM, showing the addition of genetic testing to be almost cost saving compared with clinical screening alone.[23,24]

VARIANT INTERPRETATION

Although cascade testing of family members has significant value, gathering sufficient evidence to confidently assign causative status to variants identified during proband genetic testing is a challenge. The difficulties lie with the vast amount of uncertainty inherent to this rapidly moving field, and the potential for serious harms should a variant be inappropriately used in the family. To understand this, it is important to consider the nature of genetic test results, which rather than being a binary yes or no outcome involve weighing up the evidence at a point in time. The authors use a continuum of probabilities to represent a level of confidence that a variant is not the cause (benign/likely benign) or is the cause (likely pathogenic/pathogenic). Where there is insufficient or contradictory evidence, the variant is termed uncertain, or variant of uncertain significance.

One big leap forward in the field in recent times is the standardization of variant interpretation criteria. In 2015, the American College of Medical Genetics and Genomics (ACMG) and the Association of Medical Pathologists released a joint statement on the interpretation of sequence variants,[25] and these have been widely adopted. With encouragement to further refine these for disease or gene-specific settings, these will become even more useful. The Cardiovascular Clinical Domain Working Group of the Clinical Genome Resource (Clin Gen) has recently adapted these criteria for classifying *MYH7* variants found in patients with HCM.[26] Although disease-specific modifications are useful, the general principles of the ACMG criteria encourage greater stringency. Key criteria include absence or relative rarity in large population databases, reports of the variant occurring in multiple unrelated individuals with consistent phenotypes, segregation of the variant with affected relatives, loss-of-function variants in genes where this is an established mechanism of disease, and robust functional studies demonstrating a deleterious effect. Careful evaluation and weighing of the evidence is necessary, and despite best efforts there is a subjective element to the process. Discordance between laboratories has been previously reported in numerous studies.[27–30] Key reasons for this include inconsistency in use of the ACMG criteria and lack of public sharing of important variant information, meaning some laboratories have access to information whereas others do not. Public repositories of curated variant information can help to avoid the latter situation, including ClinVar,[31] which has become an integral component of variant curation efforts.

RECLASSIFICATION

The probabilistic nature of genetic test results, where evidence is weighed to give a likelihood that a variant is causative, means that as information and knowledge change over time, so do variant classifications. Periodic reclassification of variants is an important part of the genetic testing process,[32] although there is little guidance around how this can be feasibly performed. Whether a laboratory, ordering clinician, or family are responsible for ensuring reassessment of the variant is performed periodically remains to be elucidated, and the solution likely varies depending on the clinical setting. For example, in a specialized multidisciplinary clinic, there may be capacity for cardiac genetic counselors to periodically reclassify variants prior to patients returning for their annual follow-up.

CARDIAC GENETIC COUNSELING

The role of cardiac genetic counseling, and cardiac genetic counselors specifically, has emerged as a critical part of the process of genetic testing. In general genetics, genetic counseling involves providing education, discussion of family history and inheritance risks, genetic testing options, and providing support.[33] Cardiac genetic counselors however, are uniquely subspecialized, based largely on the distinct patient population they serve. The authors have previously discussed many of the genetic counseling issues pertinent to families with inherited cardiomyopathies[34] and, in this article, focus on those relevant during the process of genetic testing.

Family History and Inheritance Risks

A detailed family history is the cornerstone of genetic medicine and can provide clinically significant information that guides many management decisions. It also offers an opportunity for the cardiac genetic counselor to develop a rapport with a patient and develop an understanding of the family dynamics and social circumstances. The family history can inform whether there is evidence of familial inheritance and the phenotype spectrum, which sometimes is more evident when considering the family as a whole. The mode of inheritance demonstrated may help interpret rare variants being assessed for causation, for example, a rare variant in the *GLA* gene identified in a patient with HCM, may indicate the well-described but rare phenocopy Fabry disease. Unlike sarcomere genes, Fabry disease is due to a deficiency of the enzyme α-galactosidase A and importantly is X-linked. A family history demonstrating male-to-male inheritance of disease would, therefore, rule out any further investigation of this variant. Other important phenocopies are shown in **Table 2**. Segregation studies can also add valuable information in families where there are multiple affected relatives who are agreeable to providing clinical and genetic data. Demonstrating a variant has co-occurred with a disease phenotype more often than would have occurred by chance can add supportive evidence of disease causation. In most inherited cardiomyopathies, there is an appreciable rate of incomplete penetrance; therefore, this article only includes relatives who have a positive phenotype and avoids unaffected relatives, in particular those who are younger than typical disease onset.

Pre and Post Test Genetic Counseling

Specific discussion prior to ordering genetic testing and during the return of the results is considered a vital aspect of the process.[6] Key points for this include

- Genetic education, including explanation of the inheritance of the disease, what genes are, how rare genetic variants can result in familial disease, and what the process of genetic testing involves.
- Possible outcomes of genetic testing, for example, identification of variants believed to cause the phenotype, uncertain variants that may require further investigation, and in some cases not finding any variants believed to be the cause of disease. It is important to set realistic expectations about the diagnostic yield of genetic testing in different settings. For example, an older HCM proband with mild disease and no family history of disease has a less than 30% chance of causative variant identified at best.[8,9,14,35,36]

Table 2
HCM Phenocopies

Phenocopy	Phenotype Features	Gene/s	Reference/s
Fabry disease	Left ventricular hypertrophy, acroparesthesia, angiokeratomas, hypohidrosis, corneal opacity, kidney disease	GLA	Monserrat et al,[48] 2007
Danon disease	Left ventricular hypertrophy, DCM, ventricular pre-excitation, skeletal myopathy, intellectual disability	LAMP2	Arad,[49] 2017; Yang et al,[50] 2005
Noonan syndrome	Asymmetric or concentric left ventricular hypertrophy, congenital heart defects, characteristic facial features, short stature	PTPN11, RAF1, RIT1	Wilkinson et al,[51] 2012; Gelb et al,[52] 2015
PRKAG2 glycogen storage disease	Left ventricular hypertrophy, ventricular pre-excitation, supraventricular arrhythmias	PRKAG2	Arad,[53] 2005
Transthyretin amyloidosis	Left ventricular hypertrophy, peripheral neuropathy, kidney disease	TTR	Vermeer et al,[54] 2017
CACNA1C cardiomyopathy	Left ventricular hypertrophy, prolonged QT interval, congenital heart disease	CACNA1C	Boczek et al,[55] 2015

- Clinical implications to the patient and family members, including options for cascade genetic testing and recommendations for clinical surveillance.
- Reproductive options that may become available to couples when a genetic diagnosis is made, including preimplantation genetic diagnosis. This involves an additional step in the in vitro fertilization process whereby a single cell of the embryo is tested for the causative variant and only unaffected embryos are implanted back in to the mother.[37]
- Implications for insurances, which are variable depending on the health care setting.
- Possibility of secondary genetic findings, which depend on the type of test ordered. A targeted panel of genes has little chance of incidental findings compared with comprehensive exome or genome sequencing.
- Exploring feelings and assessing patients' understanding of the information presented.

Studies investigating the psychological impact of genetic testing have not revealed poor outcomes,[38,39] although these were largely performed prior to next-generation sequencing technologies, which have revolutionized the entire genetics field. Recent qualitative studies point to more subtle impacts, including unaffected HCM gene carriers who perceived themselves to have disease or made changes to their lifestyle, such as reducing their effort during exercise. Poor understanding of genetic information presented was also highlighted by Burns and colleagues,[40] where HCM probands commonly misinterpreted the impact of uncertain variants, including patients who perceive the "unusual" variant to be reflective of an atypical and more severe clinical phenotype. Effective communication is therefore key, and although a primary focus of the genetic counseling process, in light of more complex genetic results, developing tools and resources to support clearer understanding is vital.[41,42]

POSTMORTEM MOLECULAR AUTOPSY AFTER SUDDEN CARDIAC DEATH IN THE YOUNG

Sudden cardiac death of a young person is a tragic complication of a variety of underlying genetic heart diseases. Although postmortem investigation can identify the cause of death in a majority of sudden cardiac deaths in the young, the death remains unexplained in up to 40% of cases.[22] Inherited cardiac arrhythmia syndromes, such as long QT syndrome, are associated with a structurally normal heart and are presumed the underlying cause in sudden unexplained cardiac death. Inherited cardiomyopathies account for 16% of sudden cardiac death in those aged less than or equal to 35 years.[22] The molecular autopsy, that is, proband genetic testing performed on postmortem DNA, can be a valuable addition over postmortem investigation alone, potentially allowing clarification of the cause of death and providing a tool for risk stratification of family members.[43]

After sudden cardiac death of a young person, a family history and premorbid medical history should be obtained, with a focus on identifying cardiac disease. Postmortem examination by a pathologist or medical examiner should include macroscopic and histologic evaluation of the heart and other organs. Genetic testing of the deceased may be the only opportunity to confirm a cause of death; thus, obtaining a postmortem blood sample is recommended[6] and mandated in several countries. If genetic heart disease is determined the cause of death, concurrent with clinical evaluation of first-degree relatives, the molecular autopsy should focus on finding a disease-causing variant in a clinically relevant gene (**Fig. 2**). For sudden unexplained deaths, genetic testing should include key cardiac arrhythmia genes[6] whereas focusing on specific cardiomyopathy gene panels is recommended where a diagnosis of an inherited cardiomyopathy is made.

Relatives of a young sudden cardiac death victim are at increased risk of psychological morbidity[44] and finding a causative variant may help a family come to terms with the uncertainty about the cause of death and the genetic risk to other relatives. The impact of uncertain findings in this setting is unclear, however. Genetic testing in families after sudden cardiac death in the young should be performed in specialist centers with multidisciplinary expertise and ideally input from a clinical psychologist.[45]

MINIMIZING POTENTIAL HARMS

There is no doubt that genetic testing for inherited cardiomyopathies can be a valuable addition to management. With all new technologies, however, comes potential for harms and/or costs to outweigh the perceived benefits. Low-value health care was predicted to have cost the United States health care system between $158 billion and $226 billion in 2011.[46] Careful attention at certain points of the genetic testing process seeks to ensure the best possible outcomes. These have been previously reviewed by Ingles and colleagues,[47] and key points are listed:

1. Choose the right genetic test: overly comprehensive genetic tests may seem a better option; however, with increasing numbers of genes sequenced comes a greater likelihood of uncertain or secondary genetic findings. In cases of a clear diagnosis, targeted genetic testing as a first-tier approach is reasonable.
2. Periodic re-evaluation of genetic findings: because the field of genetics moves quickly, processes that ensure variants are routinely re-evaluated using the latest information and

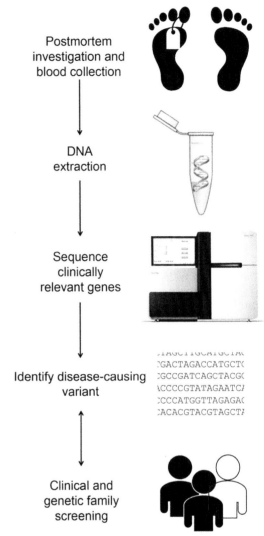

Postmortem investigation and blood collection

DNA extraction

Sequence clinically relevant genes

Identify disease-causing variant

Clinical and genetic family screening

Fig. 2. Molecular autopsy evaluation after sudden cardiac death.[56] Postmortem investigation of sudden cardiac death in the young should aim to establish whether the cause of death is due to genetic heart disease. Collection of postmortem blood allows a molecular autopsy of clinically relevant genes to identify a disease-causing DNA variant that may confirm the cause of death and be useful for the clinical management of relatives. Concurrent clinical evaluation of family members may guide the genetic testing.

variant interpretation criteria are critical. Should information about a variant change, leading to a reclassification, then having had good pretest genetic counseling makes discussion with a family less challenging.
3. Reasonable investigation of uncertain variants: decisions that clinicians make to further investigate a potential phenotype based on a dubious gene result influence the "value" of genetic testing. For example, if a patient with HCM is

found to have an uncertain variant in an inherited arrhythmia syndrome gene, such as KCNQ1, over-investigation of the patient and family members with long QT specific cardiac tests is likely unnecessary. If all uncertain variants are investigated to this extent, then the value of genetic testing very quickly is lost among the cost of unnecessary cardiac tests and leads to undue worry for the family. It is important to seek advice from centers with cardiac genetic expertise before acting on uncertain variants.

4. Expertise of a multidisciplinary clinic is the ideal model of care: given the challenges highlighted in this review, the experience of a specialized multidisciplinary team is invaluable in ensuring the best possible outcomes for families after cardiac genetic testing.

FUTURE DIRECTIONS

So much has been learned in recent years about the underlying genetics of inherited cardiomyopathies. Although the benefit to at-risk family members has always been considered the key utility of cardiac genetic testing, there is growing research to suggest genetics may someday play a role in prognosis and treatment of patients with disease. The move to a more precision-based approach to care may mean a better ability to delineate those at greatest risk of poor cardiac outcomes, including those who develop atrial fibrillation, heart failure, and sudden cardiac death. To achieve this goal, research groups worldwide need to work together, to develop large data sets that allow sufficient statistical power to elucidate these more complex associations. Although genetic testing has once been a useful adjunct to clinical management of inherited cardiomyopathies, identifying the precise genetic variant responsible for disease will become increasingly needed and potentially even a key part of management decisions.

SUMMARY

Cardiac genetic testing for inherited cardiomyopathies is available and plays an important overall role in the management of the family. The advances in the field have allowed amazing leaps forward in the tests offered and also understanding of the genetic architecture of these diseases. At present, the key benefit of genetic testing is as a risk prediction tool for at-risk family members, potentially alleviating years of unnecessary clinical screening and worry. There are well-documented challenges of cardiac genetic testing, but by

working together ways can be found to overcome them. Care should always be taken, however, and, where possible, cardiac genetic testing performed in a specialized multidisciplinary clinic incorporating cardiology and genetics is the ideal model of care.

REFERENCES

1. Ackerman MJ. Genetic purgatory and the cardiac channelopathies: exposing the variants of uncertain/unknown significance issue. Heart Rhythm 2015;12(11):2325–31.
2. Ingles J, Semsarian C. Conveying a probabilistic genetic test result to families with an inherited heart disease. Heart Rhythm 2014;11(6):1073–8.
3. Tennessen JA, Bigham AW, O'Connor TD, et al. Evolution and functional impact of rare coding variation from deep sequencing of human exomes. Science 2012;337(6090):64–9.
4. Semsarian C, Ingles J, Maron MS, et al. New perspectives on the prevalence of hypertrophic cardiomyopathy. J Am Coll Cardiol 2015;65(12):1249–54.
5. Maron BJ, Gardin JM, Flack JM, et al. Prevalence of hypertrophic cardiomyopathy in a general population of young adults. Echocardiographic analysis of 4111 subjects in the CARDIA Study. Coronary artery risk development in (young) adults. Circulation 1995;92(4):785–9.
6. Ackerman MJ, Priori SG, Willems S, et al. HRS/EHRA expert consensus statement on the state of genetic testing for the channelopathies and cardiomyopathies this document was developed as a partnership between the Heart Rhythm Society (HRS) and the European Heart Rhythm Association (EHRA). Heart Rhythm 2011;8(8):1308–39.
7. Watkins H, Ashrafian H, Redwood C. Inherited cardiomyopathies. N Engl J Med 2011;364(17): 1643–56.
8. Ingles J, Burns C, Bagnall RD, et al. Non-familial hypertrophic cardiomyopathy: prevalence, natural history, and clinical implications. Circ Cardiovasc Genet 2017;10(2) [pii:e001620].
9. Ko C, Arscott P, Concannon M, et al. Genetic testing impacts the utility of prospective familial screening in hypertrophic cardiomyopathy through identification of a nonfamilial subgroup. Genet Med 2018; 20(1):69–75.
10. Bhonsale A, Te Riele A, Sawant AC, et al. Cardiac phenotype and long-term prognosis of arrhythmogenic right ventricular cardiomyopathy/dysplasia patients with late presentation. Heart Rhythm 2017; 14(6):883–91.
11. Alcalai R, Seidman JG, Seidman CE. Genetic basis of hypertrophic cardiomyopathy: from bench to the clinics. J Cardiovasc Electrophysiol 2008;19(1): 104–10.

12. Alfares AA, Kelly MA, McDermott G, et al. CORRI-GENDUM: Results of clinical genetic testing of 2,912 probands with hypertrophic cardiomyopathy: expanded panels offer limited additional sensitivity. Genet Med 2015;17(4):319.

13. Burns C, Bagnall RD, Lam L, et al. Multiple Gene Variants in Hypertrophic Cardiomyopathy in the Era of Next-Generation Sequencing. Circ Cardiovasc Genet 2017;10(4) [pii:e001666].

14. Gruner C, Ivanov J, Care M, et al. Toronto hypertrophic cardiomyopathy genotype score for prediction of a positive genotype in hypertrophic cardiomyopathy. Circ Cardiovasc Genet 2013; 6(1):19–26.

15. Fatkin D, Seidman CE, Seidman JG. Genetics and disease of ventricular muscle. Cold Spring Harb Perspect Med 2014;4(1):a021063.

16. McNally EM, Mestroni L. Dilated cardiomyopathy: genetic determinants and mechanisms. Circ Res 2017;121(7):731–48.

17. Herman DS, Lam L, Taylor MR, et al. Truncations of titin causing dilated cardiomyopathy. N Engl J Med 2012;366(7):619–28.

18. Wolf CM, Wang L, Alcalai R, et al. Lamin A/C haploinsufficiency causes dilated cardiomyopathy and apoptosis-triggered cardiac conduction system disease. J Mol Cell Cardiol 2008;44(2):293–303.

19. Ellinor PT, MacRae CA, Thierfelder L. Arrhythmogenic right ventricular cardiomyopathy. Heart Fail Clin 2010;6(2):161–77.

20. Bhonsale A, Groeneweg JA, James CA, et al. Impact of genotype on clinical course in arrhythmogenic right ventricular dysplasia/cardiomyopathy-associated mutation carriers. Eur Heart J 2015; 36(14):847–55.

21. Castelletti S, Vischer AS, Syrris P, et al. Desmoplakin missense and non-missense mutations in arrhythmogenic right ventricular cardiomyopathy: genotype-phenotype correlation. Int J Cardiol 2017;249: 268–73.

22. Bagnall RD, Weintraub RG, Ingles J, et al. A prospective study of sudden cardiac death among children and young adults. N Engl J Med 2016;374(25):2441–52.

23. Ingles J, McGaughran J, Scuffham PA, et al. A cost-effectiveness model of genetic testing for the evaluation of families with hypertrophic cardiomyopathy. Heart 2012;98(8):625–30.

24. Wordsworth S, Leal J, Blair E, et al. DNA testing for hypertrophic cardiomyopathy: a cost-effectiveness model. Eur Heart J 2010;31(8):926–35.

25. Richards S, Aziz N, Bale S, et al. Standards and guidelines for the interpretation of sequence variants: a joint consensus recommendation of the American College of Medical Genetics and Genomics and the Association for Molecular Pathology. Genet Med 2015;17(5):405–24.

26. Kelly M, Caleshu C, Morales A, et al. Adaptation and Validation of the ACMG/AMP variant classification framework for MYH7-associated inherited cardiomyopathies: recommendations by clingen's inherited cardiomyopathy expert panel. Genet Med 2017.

27. Harrison SM, Dolinsky JS, Knight Johnson AE, et al. Clinical laboratories collaborate to resolve differences in variant interpretations submitted to ClinVar. Genet Med 2017;19(10):1096–104.

28. Yang S, Lincoln SE, Kobayashi Y, et al. CORRIGENDUM: sources of discordance among germline variant classifications in ClinVar. Genet Med 2017;19(10):1118–26.

29. Van Driest SL, Wells QS, Stallings S, et al. Association of arrhythmia-related genetic variants with phenotypes documented in electronic medical records. Jama 2016;315(1):47–57.

30. Furqan A, Arscott P, Girolami F, et al. Care in specialized centers and data sharing increase agreement in hypertrophic cardiomyopathy genetic test interpretation. Circ Cardiovasc Genet 2017;10(5) [pii: e001700].

31. Landrum MJ, Lee JM, Benson M, et al. ClinVar: public archive of interpretations of clinically relevant variants. Nucleic Acids Res 2016;44(D1):D862–8.

32. Das KJ, Ingles J, Bagnall RD, et al. Determining pathogenicity of genetic variants in hypertrophic cardiomyopathy: importance of periodic reassessment. Genet Med 2014;16(4):286–93.

33. Biesecker B. Goals of genetic counselling. Clin Genet 2001;60(5):323–30.

34. Ingles J, Yeates L, Semsarian C. The emerging role of the cardiac genetic counselor. Heart Rhythm 2011;8(12):1958–62.

35. Ingles J, Sarina T, Yeates L, et al. Clinical predictors of genetic testing outcomes in hypertrophic cardiomyopathy. Genet Med 2013;15(12):972–7.

36. Bos JM, Will ML, Gersh BJ, et al. Characterization of a phenotype-based genetic test prediction score for unrelated patients with hypertrophic cardiomyopathy. Mayo Clin Proc 2014;89(6):727–37.

37. Vermeesch JR, Voet T, Devriendt K. Prenatal and pre-implantation genetic diagnosis. Nat Rev Genet 2016;17(10):643–56.

38. Aatre RD, Day SM. Psychological issues in genetic testing for inherited cardiovascular diseases. Circ Cardiovasc Genet 2011;4(1):81–90.

39. Ingles J, Yeates L, O'Brien L, et al. Genetic testing for inherited heart diseases: longitudinal impact on health-related quality of life. Genet Med 2012;14: 749–52.

40. Burns C, Yeates L, Spinks C, et al. Attitudes, knowledge and consequences of uncertain genetic findings in hypertrophic cardiomyopathy. Eur J Hum Genet 2017;25(7):809–15.

41. Smagarinsky Y, Burns C, Spinks C, et al. Development of a communication aid for explaining

hypertrophic cardiomyopathy genetic test results. Pilot Feasibility Stud 2017;3:53.

42. Burns C, James C, Ingles J. Communication of genetic information to families with inherited rhythm disorders. Heart Rhythm 2017 [pii:S1547-5271(17)31364-4].

43. Lahrouchi N, Raju H, Lodder EM, et al. Utility of postmortem genetic testing in cases of sudden arrhythmic death syndrome. J Am Coll Cardiol 2017;69(17):2134–45.

44. Ingles J, Spinks C, Yeates L, et al. Posttraumatic stress and prolonged grief after the sudden cardiac death of a young relative. JAMA Intern Med 2016; 176(3):402–5.

45. Caleshu C, Kasparian NA, Edwards KS, et al. Interdisciplinary psychosocial care for families with inherited cardiovascular diseases. Trends Cardiovasc Med 2016;26(7):647–53.

46. Berwick DM, Hackbarth AD. Eliminating waste in US health care. JAMA 2012;307(14):1513–6.

47. Ingles J, Burns C, Barratt A, et al. Application of genetic testing in hypertrophic cardiomyopathy for preclinical disease detection. Circ Cardiovasc Genet 2015;8(6):852–9.

48. Monserrat L, Gimeno-Blanes JR, Marin F, et al. Prevalence of fabry disease in a cohort of 508 unrelated patients with hypertrophic cardiomyopathy. J Am Coll Cardiol 2007;50(25):2399–403.

49. Arad M. Cardiac danon disease: insights and challenges. Int J Cardiol 2017;245:211–2.

50. Yang Z, McMahon CJ, Smith LR, et al. Danon disease as an underrecognized cause of hypertrophic cardiomyopathy in children. Circulation 2005; 112(11):1612–7.

51. Wilkinson JD, Lowe AM, Salbert BA, et al. Outcomes in children with Noonan syndrome and hypertrophic cardiomyopathy: a study from the Pediatric Cardiomyopathy Registry. Am Heart J 2012;164(3):442–8.

52. Gelb BD, Roberts AE, Tartaglia M. Cardiomyopathies in Noonan syndrome and the other RASopathies. Prog Pediatr Cardiol 2015;39(1):13–9.

53. Arad M, Maron BJ, Gorham JM, et al. Glycogen storage diseases presenting as hypertrophic cardiomyopathy. N Engl J Med 2005;352(4):362–72.

54. Vermeer AMC, Janssen A, Boorsma PC, et al. Transthyretin amyloidosis: a phenocopy of hypertrophic cardiomyopathy. Amyloid 2017;24(2):87–91.

55. Boczek NJ, Ye D, Jin F, et al. Identification and functional characterization of a Novel CACNA1C-Mediated Cardiac disorder characterized by prolonged qt intervals with hypertrophic cardiomyopathy, congenital heart defects, and sudden cardiac death. Circ Arrhythm Electrophysiol 2015;8(5):1122–32.

56. Bagnall RD, Semsarian C. Role of the molecular autopsy in the investigation of sudden cardiac death. Prog Pediatr Cardiol 2017;45:17–23.

Genetic Pathogenesis of Hypertrophic and Dilated Cardiomyopathy

Amanda C. Garfinkel, BA[a], Jonathan G. Seidman, PhD[a],
Christine E. Seidman, MD[b,c,d],*

KEYWORDS

- Hypertrophic cardiomyopathy • Dilated cardiomyopathy • Sarcomere physiology
- Interacting-heads motif

KEY POINTS

- Diastolic dysfunction is the earliest identified biomechanical defect in human hypertrophic cardiomyopathy (HCM), whereas systolic dysfunction is the first sign of pathophysiology in dilated cardiomyopathy (DCM).
- HCM variants produce hypercontractile, poorly relaxing sarcomeres via missense mutations in sarcomere proteins.
- Titin truncating variants, yielding titin haploinsufficiency, are the most common cause of familial DCM.

INTRODUCTION

Sarcomere cardiomyopathies are genetic diseases that perturb contractile function and trigger myocardial remodeling along 2 distinct pathways. Hypertrophic cardiomyopathy (HCM) exhibits left ventricular (LV) hypertrophy with preserved systolic function and impaired relaxation. Dilated cardiomyopathy (DCM) is characterized by increased LV chamber size and systolic dysfunction. The clinical manifestations associated with sarcomere cardiomyopathies, including age of onset, severity and progression of morphologic and hemodynamic abnormalities, patient symptoms, and adverse outcomes, are highly variable: a complexity that likely reflects considerable heterogeneity of causal genes and allelic variants, and the influences of background genotypes, environmental exposures, and lifestyles. Together these factors complicate the interpretation of how particular gene mutations alter cardiac physiology.

The discovery of molecular causes for HCM and DCM has propelled gene-based diagnosis and the identification of young mutation-carriers without overt manifestations of cardiomyopathy. These "genotype-positive, phenotype-negative" individuals, although lacking hypertrophy or dilatation, exhibit cardiac abnormalities that provide insights into the earliest biomechanical defects[1–3] that link pathogenic genotypes to cardiac dysfunction.

Disclosure Statement: C.E. Seidman and J.G. Seidman are founders of, and own shares in, Myokardia Inc, a startup company that is developing therapeutics that target the sarcomere. This work was supported by grants from the National Institutes of Health (CES and JGS, 5R01HL080494, 5R01HL084553), Howard Hughes Medical Institute (CES) and The Sarnoff Foundation (AG).
a Department of Genetics, Harvard Medical School, New Research Building Room 256, 77 Avenue Louis Pasteur, Boston, MA 02115, USA; b Department of Medicine, Brigham and Women's Hospital, Harvard Medical School, 75 Francis Street, Boston, MA 02115, USA; c Department of Genetics, Brigham and Women's Hospital, Harvard Medical School, New Research Building Room 256, 77 Avenue Louis Pasteur, Boston, MA 02115, USA; d Howard Hughes Medical Institute, 4000 Jones Bridge Road, Chevy Chase, MD 20815, USA
* Corresponding author. Department of Genetics, Harvard Medical School, New Research Building Room 256, 77 Avenue Louis Pasteur, Boston, MA 02115.
E-mail address: cseidman@genetics.med.harvard.edu

Heart Failure Clin 14 (2018) 139–146
https://doi.org/10.1016/j.hfc.2017.12.004
1551-7136/18/© 2018 The Authors. Published by Elsevier Inc. This is an open access article under the CC BY-NC-ND license (http://creativecommons.org/licenses/by-nc-nd/4.0/).

Understanding these early molecular pathophysiologic events can illuminate modifiable pathways to reduce the emergence of overt HCM and DCM and limit adverse patient outcomes. In this review, the authors outline current understandings of how normal sarcomere structure and function are altered by human mutations that cause HCM or DCM.

PROPERTIES OF NORMAL SARCOMERE STRUCTURE AND FUNCTION
Components of the Cardiac Sarcomere

The sarcomere is the basic contractile unit of striated muscle, composed of thick and thin filaments (**Fig. 1**). Sarcomeres are aligned through Z-discs located at the boundary of each sarcomere and interconnected through particular thick filaments to form muscle fibers. Combined with electrophysiologic machinery, sarcomeres are responsible for contraction and relaxation of all muscle cells.

Sarcomere thin filaments are composed of α-actin (*ACTC1*) filaments and the calcium-sensitive troponin-tropomyosin regulatory apparatus, which includes troponin T (*TNNT2*), troponin I (*TNNI3*), troponin C (*TNNC1*), and α-tropomyosin (*TPM1*).

Sarcomere thick filaments contain proteins with both motor and regulatory functions. Cardiac β-myosin heavy chain (*MYH7*), the molecular motor of the thick filament, contains structural and functional domains. Myosin α-helical tails pack together to form a cylindrical backbone of thick filaments, from which pairs of myosin heads project laterally in a helical fashion at regular intervals. These protruding globular heads (denoted S1) contain a nucleotide-binding pocket with adenosine triphosphate (ATP) hydrolase activity, actin-binding sites, and regulatory domains that interact with the regulatory and essential light chains (RLC and ELC, encoded by *MYL2* and *MYL3* genes, respectively). An S2 fragment links the S1 head to myosin's tail backbone and binds myosin binding protein C (cMyBP-C, encoded by *MYBPC3*) and titin (*TTN*).[4] cMyBP-C binds actin filaments and myosin S2; these interactions are modulated

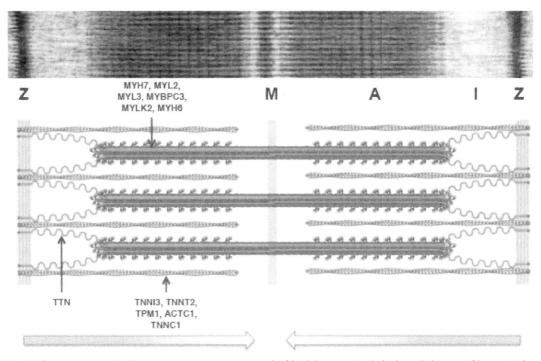

Fig. 1. The sarcomere. Cardiac sarcomeres are composed of highly organized thick and thin myofilaments that produce bands that are visible by microscopy (*top image*). One sarcomere encompasses the region between 2 Z bands, where titin and thin filaments are anchored and interact with other Z-disc proteins. The I band denotes the region lacking thick filament motor proteins that reside in the A band. The M band is an overlap region that interconnects thick filament proteins within each sarcomere. Each titin molecule spans from the Z disc to the M band, encompassing one-half of a sarcomere. The thick filament fulfills motor and regulatory functions through proteins much as cardiac β-myosin heavy chain (*MYH7*) and myosin binding protein C (*MYBPC3*). The thin filament system contains actin as well as the troponin-tropomyosin calcium-regulatory apparatus that enables and regulates actomyosin interactions. Titin(*TTN*) plays multiple roles in sarcomere function, stability, and regulation.

by phosphorylation. Dephosphorylated cMyBP-C limits thick filament sliding and thereby functions as a brake on sarcomere contractility.

Titin is the largest human protein, containing approximately 35,000 amino acids and spanning one-half of a sarcomere, from the Z disc to the central M line (see **Fig. 1**). Titin has 4 functional domains[5]: the amino-terminal Z disc participates in myofibril assembly and stabilization; an I band acts as a bidirectional spring, providing passive tension that limits sarcomere stretch in early diastole and elasticity to restore resting sarcomere length after contraction; an A band that binds myosin S1 and cMyBP-C[6] and may participate in biomechanical sensing; and a kinase-containing M band that may function in strain-sensitive signaling.[7] *TTN* encodes multiple titin isoforms: 2 with variable I band lengths due to alternative splicing are highly expressed in the heart. The longer N2BA isoform provides more elasticity, whereas the shorter N2B isoform provides more passive stiffness.[8,9]

Sarcomere Contraction

Contraction of the sarcomere occurs through actin and myosin (eg, actomyosin) interactions, through a chemomechanical cycle that begins when ATP binds to an actin-bound myosin head, causing myosin dissociation from the actin filament. Myosin ATPase then hydrolyzes ATP, prompting the myosin head's converter domain to change shape, enabling the myosin head to adopt a pre–power stroke conformation. Release of the P_i hydrolytic product facilitates myosin head rebinding at a new position along the actin filament, and a myosin power stroke produces sarcomere shortening and muscle contraction. Finally, myosin releases its adenosine 5′-diphosphate hydrolytic product, allowing new ATP binding and continued sarcomere shortening.[10]

This chemomechanical contractile apparatus is regulated by the thin filament's calcium-responsive troponin-tropomyosin complex. At low myofilament calcium concentrations, myosin-binding sites along actin filaments are sterically inhibited by tropomyosin. Upon myocyte stimulation by an action potential, an influx of calcium from the sarcoplasmic reticulum promotes calcium binding to the troponin-C unit of a troponin complex. In turn, conformational changes in the troponin-I and troponin-T subunits facilitate release of tropomyosin-based steric inhibition, allowing thin and thick filaments to interact. Importantly, this calcium regulatory system acts in a length-dependent fashion, with elongated sarcomeres exhibiting increased calcium sensitivity such that sarcomeres stretched during diastole are driven to contract upon initiation of an action potential.

Although the troponin-tropomyosin system is the major gatekeeper of the calcium-based regulation of contractility, excitation-triggered contraction depends on a complex calcium cycling system that is reviewed elsewhere.[11] Both cMyBP-C and titin participate in this calcium regulatory system: cMyBP-C phosphorylation increases myofilament calcium sensitivity, and at short sarcomere lengths, titin reduces the length-dependence of the calcium regulatory system so as to enable shorter sarcomeres to participate in the chemomechanical cycle.[12]

Although the discussion above describes contractility in terms of single actomyosin interactions, the overall power output by sarcomeres reflects the ensemble force generated by all actomyosin interactions at a given time.

Sarcomere Relaxation

At low myofilament calcium concentrations, tropomyosin-mediated steric inhibition of myosin binding sites precludes actomyosin interaction and results in sarcomere relaxation. However, relaxation is an active process with distinct structural conformations of myosins and rates of ATP hydrolysis.

Cryoelectron microscopy studies show that relaxed heads of paired myosin molecules interact through an interacting-heads motif (IHM). These interactions are dynamic and asymmetric, in that one or both of the paired myosin heads can interact with thick filament backbones, inhibit ATPase activity, and limit the potential for actomyosin interactions that generate force.[13–15] Two distinct structures of paired and relaxed myosins have been identified, each associated with different rates of energy consumption (**Fig. 2**). The disordered relaxed (DRX) state occurs when one myosin head interacts with the thick filament backbone, resulting in steric inhibition of its ATPase, whereas its partner myosin retains ATP hydrolysis activity and the potential for actomyosin interactions and force production. The superrelaxed (SRX) state occurs when both myosin heads dock onto the thick filament backbone, inhibiting ATP hydrolysis and withdrawing both myosins from thin filament interaction and force production. These IHM structures are supported by myosin interactions with the ELC and RLC that serve as scaffolding. Based on myosins' interactions with cMyBP-C and titin, these proteins are also expected to support and modulate IHM structures.

The structures and biophysical activities of sarcomeres throughout the cardiac cycle predict

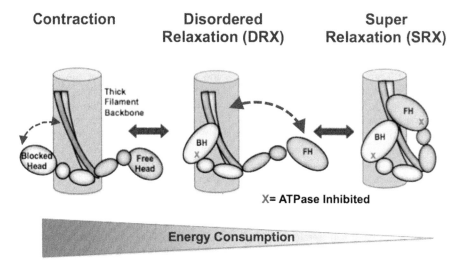

Contraction	Disordered Relaxation (DRX)	Super Relaxation (SRX)

X= ATPase Inhibited

Energy Consumption

Fig. 2. A schematic of sarcomere conformations and associated energy consumption throughout the cardiac cycle. A pair of myosin molecules is depicted, with each head denoted as blocked (BH) or free (FH). During contraction, both the BH and the FH are available for actomyosin interactions and ATP hydrolysis. During relaxation, myosins assume 2 dynamic and asymmetric conformations through the myosin IHM. In disordered relaxation (DRX), one myosin head is bound onto the thick filament backbone and is unavailable for actomyosin interactions. Energy consumption is at an intermediate level during DRX. In SRX, both myosin heads are docked onto the thick filament and energy conservation is maximized because both myosin ATPase domains are inhibited.

3 levels of energy consumption (see **Fig. 2**): contraction, with active actomyosin interactions producing power and highest rates of ATP hydrolysis; DRX with limited actomyosin interactions and intermediate rates of ATP hydrolysis; and SRX without actomyosin interactions and lowest rates of ATP hydrolysis. In later discussion, the authors show how these fundamental insights inform the mechanisms by which sarcomere gene mutations cause cardiomyopathies.

HYPERTROPHIC CARDIOMYOPATHY: A DISEASE OF POOR SARCOMERE RELAXATION

HCM is a common monogenic heart muscle disease that is clinically identified in an estimated 1 in 500 adults.[16,17] Disease-causing mutations are detected in ~30% to 60% of HCM probands, with mutations in *MYH7* and *MYBPC3* accounting for 75% of cases with an identifiable pathogenic variant.[16,17] Mutations in 6 other sarcomere genes, including *MYL2*, *MYL3*, *TPM1*, *TNNT2*, *TNNI3*, and *ACTC1*, are identified in less than 10% of cases.[17–19]

Echocardiography of patients with overt HCM and genotype-positive, phenotype-negative individuals typically reveal hyperdynamic ventricular contraction.[1] Experimental in vitro studies provide a plausible molecular explanation for these clinical observations: sarcomere proteins or isolated myofibrils with HCM mutations have increased power production.[17–19] Experimental studies also indicate

that hyperdynamic contraction may be an essential mediator of the cardiac remodeling in HCM. To study the effects of attenuating hyperdynamic contraction, researchers performed a small molecule screen that identified MYK-461, an allosteric inhibitor of myosin ATPase that reduced fractional shortening of cardiomyocytes in a dose-dependent manner. Oral administration of MYK-461 to prehypertrophic mice harboring pathogenic HCM mutations in myosin (R403Q, R453C, or R719W) normalized contractility in a dose-dependent fashion and attenuated development of LV hypertrophy and fibrosis.[20] These observations also indicate a window of opportunity in which restoration of physiologic sarcomere performance might prevent cardiac remodeling.

However, hypercontractility and increased sarcomere power alone are unlikely to fully explain how mutations cause HCM pathophysiology. First, all HCM mutations in myosin encode a single amino acid substitution, and it is extremely unlikely that each of these bolster rather than depress sarcomere performance. Second, increased contractility fails to explain diastolic dysfunction of HCM, a predominant pathophysiologic abnormality that drives patients' symptoms and adverse outcomes. Third, diastolic dysfunction is an early HCM abnormality that is demonstrable even in genotype-positive, phenotype-negative individuals.[1]

These data prompted consideration of whether HCM mutations fundamentally perturb relaxation as well as sarcomere contraction. This question was addressed by determining if the location of HCM missense variants in *MYH7*, *MYL2*, and *MYL3* were predicted to alter IHM interactions that occur during sarcomere relaxation.[4] Among 6112 HCM patients studied, 78% of *MYH7* pathogenic mutations and all 4 ELC and RLC pathogenic mutations altered IHM-interacting residues and amino acid charges. These findings predict that HCM mutations would destabilize IHM interactions and as a consequence diminish the proportions of myosins in the SRX state while increasing myosins in the DRX state, which enable actomyosin interactions ATP hydrolysis.[4]

cMyBP-C is proposed to stabilize the IHM.[4] Because HCM mutations in cMyBP-C reduce its levels, these should also destabilize the IHM. Recent experimental data confirm this model: human and mouse hearts with *MYBPC3* mutations show significantly reduced SRX and increased DRX.[21,22]

Together, these biophysical data provide a compelling explanation for preclinical[1–3] findings and overt HCM pathophysiology,[23] including hyperdynamic contractility from augmented motor properties and increased DRX, diastolic dysfunction from reduced levels of the SRX, and excessive energy consumption from both. The hypothesis that sarcomere hypercontractility in HCM is a secondary effect of IHM-destabilizing mutations, rather than a primary effect of the mutations themselves, is logical from a conceptual perspective, resolving the idiosyncratic supposition that sarcomere proteins are somehow functionally enhanced by HCM mutations.

Although HCM-linked mutations in thick filament proteins thus disrupt sarcomere physiology through direct interference with components of the actomyosin system and the IHM, hypercontractility and diastolic dysfunction can also be produced indirectly via disruption of the sarcomere's calcium-based regulatory system. At low calcium concentrations, such as those seen in LV cardiomyocytes during diastole, tropomyosin inhibits actin interactions with myosin and thereby contributes to relaxation. However, experimental models of HCM-linked mutations in tropomyosin (*TPM1*) and troponin complex subunits (*TNNC1*, *TNNI3*, *TNNT2*) have consistently shown myofibrillar hypersensitivity to calcium, implying a failure to block sarcomere shortening at concentrations normally associated with relaxation.[24,25] cMyBP-C also plays a role in the calcium regulatory system of the sarcomere, and increased calcium sensitivity also appears to be a driving pathophysiologic mechanism in *MYBPC3*-linked HCM.[26] This appears to be an indirect mechanism because calcium sensitivity in human HCM specimens is

normalized by protein kinase A-mediated correction of troponin I dephosphorylation.[27,28]

Increased calcium sensitivity has also been observed in analyses of multiple human HCM samples,[28] perhaps indicating that this may be a shared response to HCM sarcomere mutations. Calcium abnormalities also contribute to clinical phenotypes. For example, a *TPM1* founder mutation in the Finnish population causes HCM with more arrhythmias than other HCM mutations.[25] However, calcium dysregulation is unlikely to be the primary defect, as mutations in calcium regulatory proteins cause arrhythmic disorders with minimal or no hypertrophy.

In summary, HCM mutations have multiple distinct mechanisms that disrupt sarcomere properties and produce a common molecular phenotype of hyperdynamic contractility, poor relaxation, and increased energy consumption. These fundamental pathophysiologic anomalies are manifested early in preclinical genotype-positive, phenotype-negative individuals and drive hypertrophic remodeling that produces overt HCM.

DILATED CARDIOMYOPATHY: A DISEASE OF IMPAIRED SARCOMERE CONTRACTION

DCM is a prevalent disorder with many causes that span from acquired toxic and metabolic insults to sarcomere gene mutations. Monogenic causes contribute to 25% to 50% of all DCM cases,[29] and among these, *TTN* mutations predominate. Truncating mutations in *TTN* (TTNtvs) occur in 25% of end-stage disease and in 15% of ambulatory DCM patients.[7,8] DCM mutations in other sarcomere genes, including *MYH7*, *MYBPC3*, *TNNT2*, and *TPM1*, alter different residues than mutations that cause HCM and are far less common.[30] Systolic dysfunction is the hallmark pathophysiologic feature of DCM and is also demonstrable in genotype-positive, phenotype-negative individuals. Reduced sarcomere contractility can increase ventricular volumes to maintain cardiac output through the Frank-Starling mechanism, producing the thin-walled LV appearance that is observed in overt DCM.[31]

Analyses of myosins with DCM mutations demonstrate opposite biophysical properties than myosin mutations that cause HCM. DCM mutations are concentrated in the nucleotide-binding pocket and impair ATP hydrolysis and actomyosin interactions to decrease sarcomere power.[32] Unlike HCM mutations, myosin DCM mutations rarely alter amino acids involved in IHM interactions; as such, these variants have minimal impact on sarcomere relaxation.[4] Troponin mutations also cause DCM by altering different residues than those that cause HCM. Moreover, in contrast to the increased calcium sensitivity seen that occurs in HCM *TNNT2* mutations, DCM mutations reduce myofibrillar calcium sensitivity in vitro and may enhance tropomyosin blockade of actomyosin at calcium concentrations that should promote sarcomere shortening.[24] Although these findings explain how *TNNT2* and *MYH7* mutations reduce sarcomere contractility and systolic function in DCM, these mechanisms do not directly involve titin nor explain how TTNtvs, the most common genetic cause of DCM, cause disease.

Titin is encoded by 364 exons, and many of these harbor many rare sequence variants. Based on analyses of the general population, most individuals have at least 23 variable amino acids in titin and 2% carry a rare TTNtv that foreshortens the molecule,[8,17] most of which do not cause disease. Studies of human heart tissues and human cardiomyocytes derived from induced pluripotent stem cells (hiPSC-CM) with TTNtvs identified in healthy individuals indicate that tolerated mutations are excluded from both major cardiac titin isoforms by alternative splicing of exons.[8] By contrast, TTNtvs that cause DCM are within constitutively expressed exons of the N2BA and N2B titin isoforms.[8,33]

TTNtvs that cause DCM are more highly enriched in the A band.[7–9] Indeed, a recent meta-analysis of greater than 2400 DCM cases and greater than 61,000 controls showed that A-band TTNtvs are profoundly associated with DCM (odds ratio = 49.8), whereas TTNtvs in other constitutively expressed exons conveyed lower risks for DCM (odds ratio = 5.3–32.0).[34] Although the exclusion of TTNtvs due to alternative splicing of exons may explain why these are unlikely to cause DCM, current understanding of A-band enrichment of TTNtvs in DCM remains rudimentary.[33]

The cumulative evidence from analyses of human cardiac transcriptomes and proteomes and functional studies of hiPSC-CM and rodent models indicates that TTNtvs cause haploinsufficiency of titin.[33] hiPSC-CM with heterozygous TTNtv have 50% of normal titin levels and diminished sarcomere content and organization, whereas hiPSC-CM with homozygous TTNtvs express no titin and lack almost all sarcomeres.[33] These data, coupled with the early developmental expression of titin when primordial cells adopt a cardiomyocyte fate, support the conclusion that titin is critical for sarcomere assembly and that titin levels correlate with sarcomere content. TTNtv could result in fewer sarcomeres and thereby account for inadequate cardiac responses to stresses, such as adrenergic stimulation and

hemodynamic load. Consistent with this model, TTNtvs have been identified in women with peripartum cardiomyopathy, an enigmatic form of DCM that occurs in the late stages of pregnancy or postpartum.[35]

TTNtv may also reduce passive stiffness in the heart. Passive stiffness in isolated cardiac myofibrils from DCM patients with mutations in *TTN*, *TNNI3*, *TNNC1*, and *MYH7* was on average 38% lower than in control specimens.[29] Myofibrils with mutations in sarcomere proteins excepting titin also had additional biomechanical deficits, including faster rates of fiber relaxation; these were not observed with TTNtvs. A reduction in the heart's passive stiffness early in diastole would lead to excessive sarcomere stretch, reducing the overlap of actin and myosin filaments and decreasing sarcomere shortening during systole.

Reduced passive tension in cardiomyocytes with TTNtv may relate to titin's role in sarcomere assembly and maintenance. The titin A band contains a C zone with 11 superrepeat elements that bind myosin and cMyBP-C. Each superrepeat element is ∼43-nm long, the same length as the interval at which myosin head pairs protrude from the thick filament.[36] This finding has led to the hypothesis that the C zone in titin's A band determines thick filament length, an important parameter of contractility. The observation that hiPSCs-CMs with TTNtv in the A band develop abnormal, irregular sarcomeres supports this model.[33] In addition, a recently developed mouse model that lacks the first 2 C-zone superrepeats resulted in shorter thick filament lengths and generated less force than did normal mice.[37] Together these data indicate that reduced sarcomere force due to TTNtv reflects impaired sarcomerogenesis and reduced passive myofibrillar tension.

There is still much more to learn about how TTNtvs cause DCM, including the roles of environmental factors in triggering cardiac decompensation. DCM caused by TTNtv typically occurs after middle age,[28,33] and TTNtvs are very uncommon in DCM that presents during childhood.[38] In addition to promoting peripartum cardiomyopathy, TTNtv may contribute to other acquired forms of DCM, including in patients with anthracycline-induced cardiomyopathy.[39] Together these observations indicate that by impairing sarcomerogenesis, TTNtvs limit the heart's compensatory responses to a wide range of physiologic and environmental stresses.

In summary, DCM mutations in genes that encode sarcomere proteins reduce the performance of the contractile apparatus. Mutations in titin are particularly impactful because of their high prevalence in many forms of DCM and because these reduce sarcomere content. Disruption of sarcomere function and/or structure causes the systolic dysfunction that characterizes DCM.

CONCLUSIONS AND FUTURE DIRECTIONS

Recent years have seen meaningful growth in the understanding of the molecular-level pathophysiology that informs how sarcomere gene mutations cause HCM and DCM. HCM mutations produce deficits in sarcomere relaxation, whereas DCM mutations disturb force generation. These advances also raise many unanswered questions. Future studies are needed to discern how cMyBP-C mutations, a prevalent cause of HCM, alter sarcomere relaxation, whether the many titin missense variants contribute to unsolved cases of DCM, and if additional sarcomere proteins, particularly the RLC and ELC, influence biophysical properties of the sarcomere in health and disease. The combination of hiPSC technologies and genetic engineering provides unparalleled opportunities to answer these questions and to discover how other human mutations perturb sarcomere structure and function. The authors anticipate that deeper understanding of these mechanistic features will complement gene-based diagnosis by defining strategies to modulate the sarcomere so as to limit or prevent HCM and DCM.

REFERENCES

1. Ho CY, Sweitzer NK, McDonough B, et al. Assessment of diastolic function with Doppler tissue imaging to predict genotype in preclinical hypertrophic cardiomyopathy. Circulation 2002;105(25):2992–7.
2. Ashrafian H, McKenna WJ, Watkins H. Disease pathways and novel therapeutic targets in hypertrophic cardiomyopathy. Circ Res 2011;109(1): 86–96.
3. Ashrafian H, Redwood C, Blair E, et al. Hypertrophic cardiomyopathy: a paradigm for myocardial energy depletion. Trends Genet 2003;19(5):263–8.
4. Alamo L, Ware JS, Pinto A, et al. Effects of myosin variants on interacting-heads motif explain distinct hypertrophic and dilated cardiomyopathy phenotypes. Elife 2017;6. https://doi.org/10.7554/eLife.24634.
5. Henderson CA, Gomez CG, Novak SM, et al. Overview of the muscle cytoskeleton. Compr Physiol 2017;7(3):891–944.
6. Kontrogianni-Konstantopoulos A, Ackermann MA, Bowman AL, et al. Muscle giants: molecular scaffolds in sarcomerogenesis. Physiol Rev 2009;89(4): 1217–67.
7. Herman DS, Lam L, Taylor MR, et al. Truncations of titin causing dilated cardiomyopathy. N Engl J Med 2012;366(7):619–28.
8. Roberts AM, Ware JS, Herman DS, et al. Integrated allelic, transcriptional, and phenomic dissection of the cardiac effects of titin truncations in health and disease. Sci Transl Med 2015;7(270):270ra6.
9. Gerull B. The rapidly evolving role of titin in cardiac physiology and cardiomyopathy. Can J Cardiol 2015;31(11):1351–9.
10. Spudich JA. Hypertrophic and dilated cardiomyopathy: four decades of basic research on muscle lead to potential therapeutic approaches to these devastating genetic diseases. Biophys J 2014;106(6): 1236–49.
11. Eisner DA, Caldwell JL, Kistamás K, et al. Calcium and excitation-contraction coupling in the heart. Circ Res 2017;121(2):181–95.
12. Muhle-Goll C, Habeck M, Cazorla O, et al. Structural and functional studies of titin's fn3 modules reveal conserved surface patterns and binding to myosin S1–a possible role in the Frank-Starling mechanism of the heart. J Mol Biol 2001;313(2):431–47.
13. Woodhead JL, Zhao F-Q, Craig R, et al. Atomic model of a myosin filament in the relaxed state. Nature 2005;436(7054):1195–9.
14. Alamo L, Wriggers W, Pinto A, et al. Three-dimensional reconstruction of tarantula myosin filaments suggests how phosphorylation may regulate myosin activity. J Mol Biol 2008;384(4):780–97.
15. Suk Jung HS, Komatsu S, Ikebe M, et al. Head–head and head–tail interaction: a general mechanism for switching off myosin II activity in cells. Mol Biol Cell 2008;19(8):3234–42.
16. Maron BJ, Gardin JM, Flack JM, et al. Prevalence of hypertrophic cardiomyopathy in a general population of young adults: echocardiographic analysis of 4111 subjects in the CARDIA study. Circulation 1995;92(4):785–9.
17. Burke MA, Cook SA, Seidman JG, et al. Clinical and mechanistic insights into the genetics of cardiomyopathy. J Am Coll Cardiol 2016;68(25):2871–86.
18. Alfares AA, Kelly MA, McDermott G, et al. Results of clinical genetic testing of 2,912 probands with hypertrophic cardiomyopathy: expanded panels offer limited additional sensitivity. Genet Med 2015; 17(11):880–8.
19. Walsh R, Thomson KL, Ware JS, et al. Reassessment of Mendelian gene pathogenicity using 7,855 cardiomyopathy cases and 60,706 reference samples. Genet Med 2017;19(2):192–203.
20. Green EM, Wakimoto H, Anderson RL, et al. A small-molecule inhibitor of sarcomere contractility suppresses hypertrophic cardiomyopathy in mice. Science 2016;351(6273):617–21.
21. McNamara JW, Li A, Smith NJ, et al. Ablation of cardiac myosin binding protein-C disrupts the super-

relaxed state of myosin in murine cardiomyocytes. J Mol Cell Cardiol 2016;94:65–71.

22. McNamara JW, Li A, Lal S, et al. MYBPC3 mutations are associated with a reduced super-relaxed state in patients with hypertrophic cardiomyopathy. PLoS One 2017;12(6):1–22.

23. Marian AJ, Braunwald E. Hypertrophic cardiomyopathy: genetics, pathogenesis, clinical manifestations, diagnosis, and therapy. Circ Res 2017; 121(7):749–70.

24. Sommese RF, Nag S, Sutton S, et al. Effects of troponin T cardiomyopathy mutations on the calcium sensitivity of the regulated thin filament and the actomyosin cross-bridge kinetics of human-cardiac myosin. PLoS One 2013;8(12):e83403.

25. Ojala M, Prajapati C, Pölönen RP, et al. Mutation-specific phenotypes in hiPSC-derived cardiomyocytes carrying either myosin-binding protein C or α-tropomyosin mutation for hypertrophic cardiomyopathy. Stem Cells Int 2016;2016:1684792.

26. Barefield D, Kumar M, de Tombe PP, et al. Contractile dysfunction in a mouse model expressing a heterozygous MYBPC3 mutation associated with hypertrophic cardiomyopathy. Am J Physiol Hear Circ Physiol 2014;306(6):H807–15.

27. Van Dijk SJ, Dooijes D, dos Remedios C, et al. Cardiac myosin-binding protein C mutations and hypertrophic cardiomyopathy: haploinsufficiency, deranged phosphorylation, and cardiomyocyte dysfunction. Circulation 2009;119(11):1473–83.

28. Sequeira V, Wijnker PJM, Nijenkamp LL, et al. Perturbed length-dependent activation in human hypertrophic cardiomyopathy with missense sarcomeric gene mutations. Circ Res 2013;112(11):1491–505.

29. Vikhorev PG, Smoktunowicz N, Munster AB, et al. Abnormal contractility in human heart myofibrils from patients with dilated cardiomyopathy due to mutations in TTN and contractile protein genes. Sci Rep 2017;7(1):14829.

30. Marian AJ, van Rooij E, Roberts R. Genetics and genomics of single-gene cardiovascular diseases: common hereditary cardiomyopathies as prototypes of single-gene disorders. J Am Coll Cardiol 2016; 68(25):2831–49.

31. Lakdawala NK, Thune JJ, Colan SD, et al. Subtle abnormalities in contractile function are an early manifestation of sarcomere mutations in dilated cardiomyopathy. Circ Cardiovasc Genet 2012;5(5): 503–10.

32. Schmitt JP, Debold EP, Ahmad F, et al. Cardiac myosin missense mutations cause dilated cardiomyopathy in mouse models and depress molecular motor function. Proc Natl Acad Sci U S A 2006; 103(6):14525–30.

33. Hinson JT, Chopra A, Nafissi N, et al. Titin mutations in iPS cells define sarcomere insufficiency as a cause of dilated cardiomyopathy. Science 2015; 349(6251):982–6.

34. Schafer S, de Marvao A, Adami E, et al. Titin-truncating variants affect heart function in disease cohorts and the general population. Nat Genet 2016; 49(1):46–53.

35. Ware JS, Li J, Mazaika E, et al. Shared genetic predisposition in peripartum and dilated cardiomyopathies. N Engl J Med 2016;374(3):233–41.

36. Furst DO, Nave R, Osborn MW, et al. Repetitive titin epitopes with a 42 nm spacing coincide in relative position with known A band striations also identified by major myosin-associated proteins. An immunoelectron-microscopical study on myofibrils. J Cell Sci 1989; 94(Pt 1):119–25.

37. Tonino P, Kiss B, Strom J, et al. The giant protein titin regulates the length of the striated muscle thick filament. Nat Commun 2017;8(1):1041.

38. Fatkin D, Lam L, Herman DS, et al. Titin truncating mutations: a rare cause of dilated cardiomyopathy in the young. Prog Pediatr Cardiol 2016;40:41–5.

39. Linschoten M, Teske AJ, Baas AF, et al. Truncating titin (TTN) variants in chemotherapy-induced cardiomyopathy. J Card Fail 2017;23(6):476–9.

Biophysical Derangements in Genetic Cardiomyopathies

Melissa L. Lynn, PhD[a], Sarah J. Lehman, PhD[b],
Jil C. Tardiff, MD, PhD[c],*

KEYWORDS

- Cardiomyopathies • Primary • Phosphorylation potential • Calcium signaling • Protein stability
- Therapeutics

KEY POINTS

- Current therapeutics aimed at symptom palliation do not address the complex heterogeneity of disease presentation in genetic cardiomyopathies.
- We discuss three proposed "bins" that provide mechanistic insight in the early and compensatory phases of cardiomyopathic progression.
- A more refined classification based on primary biophysical derangements could lead to direct interventions that target early dysregulation.

INTRODUCTION

In 1990, a landmark study established the link between a genetic mutation in the sarcomeric β-myosin heavy chain gene and hypertrophic cardiomyopathy (HCM).[1] This seminal discovery was the first time a mutation in a sarcomeric gene was causally linked to disease, thus beginning the "genetic era" of cardiomyopathies. Since then, more than 450 mutations in sarcomere-associated genes encoding thick filament-associated proteins, thin filament (TF) proteins, and titin have been implicated in the development of HCM and dilated cardiomyopathy (DCM).[2–4] The recognition of the genetic basis of cardiomyopathic remodeling was key to furthering understanding of the complex heterogeneity of disease presentation.

Although the genetic basis of cardiomyopathies is widely recognized, the link between genotype and phenotype and understanding of the precise mechanisms underlying these diseases remains unclear. To add to this disconnect, by the time patients become symptomatic, pathology has often progressed past the initial phase (when treatment would be more effective) to advanced end-stage pathology. Strikingly, despite the persistence of heart disease as a leading cause of death, over the last three decades there has been a marked decline in the innovation of cardiovascular pharmaceuticals.[5] Similarly, the only treatments currently available for HCM are indirect, used primarily for symptom palliation. Further complicating this is the oft-noted finding that similar mutations clustered in "hot spots" in sarcomeric proteins often lead to disparate phenotypes. We

Disclosure Statement: Nothing to disclose.
Funded by: National Institutes of Health (R01 HL075619 and R01 HL107046).
[a] Department of Medicine, University of Arizona, Room 317, 1656 East Mabel Street, Tucson, AZ 85724, USA;
[b] Department of Physiological Sciences, University of Arizona, Room 317, 1656 East Mabel Street, Tucson, AZ 85724, USA; [c] Department of Medicine, University of Arizona, Room 312, 1656 East Mabel Street, Tucson, AZ 85724, USA
* Corresponding author.
E-mail address: jtardiff@email.arizona.edu

and others have recently shown that to address this disconnect it is paramount to understand the primary biophysical derangements associated with individual mutations.

Given the complexity of genetic cardiomyopathies, it is perhaps more useful to characterize cardiomyopathy-causing mutations based on their primary biophysical insult rather than their late-stage pathology. Linking the biophysical insult to the earliest molecular dysregulations observed, or "binning," could lead to targeted therapies for the preclinical cohort that alter the natural progression of the disease (**Fig. 1**). This article focuses on how the molecular changes, elicited by mutations in myofilament proteins (enzymatic thick filament, myosin; and the regulatory TF, Tm, cTnC, cTnI, cTnT), trigger specific pathways that lead to cardiomyopathies. Of note, because titin mutations are largely linked to DCM and represent a particular complex array of mutations, it is not covered here. Its role in genetic cardiomyopathies is well reviewed elsewhere.[6–8]

We discuss three proposed "bins" that provide well-studied, mechanistic insight for a wide range of cardiomyopathies in the early and compensatory phase of the disease. These "bins" include

- Phosphorylation potential: Specifically, how mutations in myofilament proteins alter the ability to respond to physiologic β-adrenergic stimulation.
- Calcium homeostasis: Specifically, how mutations in myofilament proteins lead to downstream changes in calcium handling in the myocyte.
- Structural stability and flexibility: Specifically, how mutations in myofilament proteins alter intramolecular and intermolecular allostery.

PHOSPHORYLATION POTENTIAL

The basic function of the cardiovascular system is to match cardiac output to the hemodynamic demands of the body. The ability of the heart to couple input to output and respond to systemic needs on a beat-to-beat basis is tightly regulated by the autonomic nervous system.[9] At the level of the cardiac myocyte, β-adrenergic (β-AD) stimulation elicits a signaling cascade mediated by protein kinase A (PKA) phosphorylation. This culminates in increased lusitropy (relaxation) and inotropy (contractility) allowing the heart to fill more efficiently and beat more rapidly. Downstream targets of PKA phosphorylation in the cardiomyocyte include the myofilament (cTnI), sarcolemma (Na-Ca exchanger, LTCC [L-type calcium channel]), and sarcoplasmic reticulum (SR-bound Ca^{2+}-ATPase, phospholamban, ryanodine receptor). These targets work synergistically to fine tune the calcium-dependent mechanical response of the myocyte.

The normal structural response to phosphorylation is small yet the functional impact is significant. A robust example of this structure-function relationship is the phosphorylation of cTnI, the inhibitory subunit of cTn, at Ser22/23 (Ser23/24 in mice). On β-AD stimulation, PKA-mediated phosphorylation of cTnI elicits an allosteric rearrangement of cTn such that the calcium sensitivity of force development is decreased and ventricular relaxation can occur more rapidly.[10] Phosphorylation of cTnI and calcium sensitivity are intrinsically linked because the role of cTn is two-fold; it regulates the response of the sarcomere to increased demand via phosphorylation, and it is the calcium switch that initiates contraction (discussed later). A critical interface exists between the N-terminal extension of cTnI (cNTnI) and the C-lobe of cTnC that has a reduced affinity in response to PKA phosphorylation (**Fig. 2**).[12–14] This reduction in affinity of cTnI for cTnC mediates the rapid release of calcium from the N-lobe of cTnC (cNTnC) via electrostatic repulsion of cNTnI, and suboptimal repositioning of cNTnC, thus affecting calcium sensitivity.[15,16]

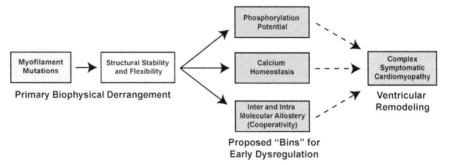

Proposed "Bins" for
Early Dysregulation

Fig. 1. Summary of cardiomyopathic disease progression and proposed "binning." *Dashed line* represents the unknown time-course of disease progression between early dysregulation and ventricular remodeling.

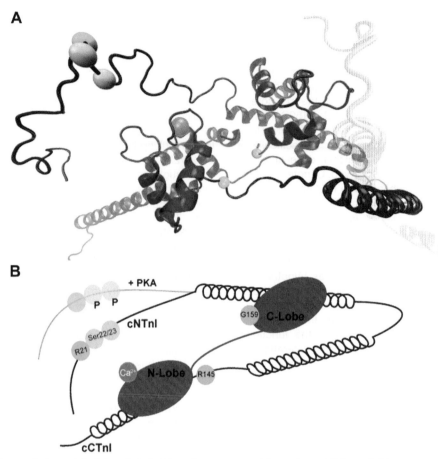

Fig. 2. (*A*) Atomistic model of the cTnI-cTnC interface generated from the publicly available average structure by JR Exequiel Pineda.[11] cTnI (*dark blue*), cTnC (*red*), cTnT (*yellow*). *Dark* versus *light* areas of the protein indicate spatial depth that is near and far, respectively. cTnT is intentionally faded for clarity. Mutation sites discussed (cTnI R21 and R145, and cTnC G159) are marked with *green beads*, cTnI Ser22/23 is highlighted with *cyan beads*, and the active calcium binding pocket is marked with a *gray bead*. (*B*) Two-dimensional representation of the interface, including the structural rearrangement on PKA phosphorylation.

Impaired response to the β-AD signaling cascade is a commonly reported finding in heart failure.[17] However, in HCM and DCM this desensitization is observed in the absence of changes in the concentration of plasma catecholamines and before the onset of heart failure.[18–20] Notably, this failure to augment contractility is often out of proportion to the degree of remodeling, where diastolic dysfunction may be present with or without hypertrophy.[21] These observations beg the question of how a single amino acid substitution within the myofilament could trigger these downstream events leading to a change in β-AD responsiveness. Because of the inherent lack of structure in "intrinsically disordered" segments of cTn, the N-terminal extension of cTnI and cTnT, among others, has been notoriously difficult to study.[22,23] Recently, molecular dynamics simulations (MDS), a powerful

computational tool for monitoring the rapid fluctuation of these flexible segments over an ensemble of conformations, have enhanced the ability to study the dynamic nature of cTn.[14,24] Thus, mutations in TF proteins that alter this critical interface could represent an early trigger, responsible for the blunted response that is out-of-proportion to the degree of remodeling. In fact, it was postulated in 1995 that targeting this interaction may be a promising approach in the treatment of heart failure.[25] Although clinical trials using levosimendan (a calcium sensitizer that binds the cTnI-cTnC interface) have demonstrated mixed results, it is not approved for use in the United States because no improvement in short- or long-term outcome beyond tradiional inotropes (ie, dobutamine) was reported.[25–29] Because of its inherent complexity, an improved understanding of the cTnI-cTnC interface is necessary to properly target interventions that directly ameliorate disruptions caused by myofilament mutations.

Clinically relevant cardiomyopathy-associated mutations have been reported in the proteins of the cTnI-cTnC interface, including cTnT, which has known effects on modulating the cTn core.[30] An illustrative example is cTnC G159D (DCM), which was shown to alter the cTnI-cTnC interface by Biesiadecki and colleagues.[31] Specifically, a blunting of the expected calcium desensitization on PKA treatment was observed. Of note, pseudo-phosphorylation, whereby the PKA-targeted sites were mutated to mimic the negatively charged phosphate ions, was also found to be insufficient to induce a decrease in calcium sensitivity.[31] These data suggest that these cTnI-PKA sites are inaccessible in the presence of cTnC-G159D. This structural rearrangement was hypothesized to lead to an increased affinity of the C-lobe of cTnC for the cNTnI, the opposite of the physiologic effect of phosphorylation of cTnI, thereby hindering the release of calcium from the functional cNTnC. This further suggests that alterations in the cTnI-cTnC interface, rather than changes in the calcium-binding pocket on cTnC, govern calcium affinity. Although illustrative, the prevalence of mutations in cTnC is low, suggesting low tolerance and that alterations at the interface are more commonly caused by allosteric effects of mutations in other myofilament proteins.

Cardiomyopathy-associated mutations in cTnI and cTnT are more common, with mutations in hot-spot regions of both proteins shown to alter β-AD signaling and some proposed to alter the cTnI-cTnC interface.[32–37] Strikingly, these mutations have similar effects on the interface as reported for cTnC-G159D despite being primarily causative for HCM. The HCM-linked cTnI-R145G mutation (R146G in rodents) has been shown to have an increased calcium-binding affinity at baseline.[34] This increase was linked to an increased cTnI-cTnC affinity that was not reduced by introduction of Ser23D/24D pseudophosphorylation.[34] These results suggest that, as previously noted, PKA is unable to decrease the affinity of cTnI for cTnC in the presence of the mutation. Similarly, cTnI-R21C has been shown to lead to a blunted response to β-AD signaling in vivo, and has demonstrated an increased cTnI-cTnC interface affinity.[34] The location of these cTnI mutations, discretely located within the N-terminus (R21C) and C-terminus (R145G), highlights the potential for allosteric propagation of structure-induced functional effects within this highly organized system. This is further highlighted in the cTnT-R92L mutation in which we have measured a myofilament-specific decrease in PKA-mediated cTnI phosphorylation in the absence of severe downstream calcium-handling abnormalities (discussed in depth later).[37] This suggests that cTnT-R92L is altering the structure of the cTn core and cTnI-cTnC interface, despite its relative distance, blocking PKA from accessing its binding site. MDS suggests that in the presence of cTnT-R92L, cNTnI is closer to cNTnC likely resulting in PKA's inability to phosphorylate Ser22/23.[11]

Although the predominant effects of mutations in this critical interface are to decrease the accessibility of Ser22/23 for PKA, there are a few exceptions. The restrictive cardiomyopathy-associated cTnI-R145W mutation has been shown to reduce the interaction frequency between the C-lobe of cTnC and cTnI, yet causes an increase in myofilament calcium sensitivity.[33] Interestingly, this increased sensitivity is opposite to what would be predicted in the face of a decreased affinity of the cTnI-cTnC interface. However, MDS predictions suggest that the significant structural alterations ultimately negate the functional impact of Ser23/24 phosphorylation.[33] These complex examples of the functional deficits induced by structural alterations underscore the need for continued research into this highly relevant interface within the cTn core.

Although regionally and pathogenically disparate, these mutations have similar effects on the phosphorylation potential of cTnI and calcium-dependent relaxation. This suggests a critical structural mechanism exists whereby cTnI-cTnC interaction regulates the response to β-AD stimulation, a regulation that can become uncoupled by pathogenic myofilament mutations. Thus, pharmacologic targeting of the interface may represent a promising area of investigation in treating the progression to heart failure in cardiomyopathies. Promising work recently demonstrated that epigallocatechin-3-gallate binds the cTnI-cTnC interface and effectively decreases calcium sensitivity maintaining the coupling of cTnI phosphorylation-dependent calcium sensitivity.[38] However, continued research is necessary to translate this therapy into the clinical realm.

CALCIUM HOMEOSTASIS

In addition to blunted response to β-AD stimulation and subsequent calcium-dependent relaxation in the heart, an extensively studied mechanism of genetic cardiomyopathy-driven disease pathogenesis is altered calcium homeostasis. This critical signaling molecule is intimately involved in excitation-contraction coupling (ECC) (reviewed in Ref.[39]). In brief, depolarization of the sarcolemma leads to the opening of voltage-gated LTCC, allowing for an influx of calcium into the myocyte. LTCC are organized in close proximity to the SR (the main intracellular calcium store) via T-tubules. Ryanodine receptor located on the membrane of the SR binds free calcium, thereby opening and raising intracellular calcium via calcium-induced calcium release. Free calcium binds to cTnC leading to cross-bridge formation and force-generation. On release of calcium from cTnC, free calcium is removed from the myocyte primarily via SR-bound Ca^{2+}-ATPase 2a, lowering free calcium to resting levels. Thus, given the role of ECC in dynamic regulation of systolic and diastolic function, and its well-described dysregulation in sudden cardiac death, the components of this system are potential targets for precise therapeutic interventions.

Many studies have described common alterations in myocellular calcium handling in HCM and DCM including prolonged calcium transients, increased resting calcium levels, and reduced SR calcium content.[40–43] However, to link these downstream changes to primary insults at the myofilament level, we must define alterations in the buffering capacity of the myofilament. An extensively studied aspect of this myofilament-calcium axis is the calcium sensitivity of force generation in myofibrils and/or reconstituted proteins. Studies have reported disease-specific alterations in force generation whereby HCM-associated mutations are described as calcium-sensitized, whereas DCM-associated mutations are described as calcium-desensitized.[44–46] Of note, although the dysregulation in calcium-sensitivity is proposed to be a secondary mechanism in disease progression, the subsequent downstream alterations in myocellular calcium handling are posited to have differential roles in pathogenesis. Specifically, the increased calcium transients and peak amplitude of calcium seen in multiple models of DCM suggest a maintained ECC pathway where the downstream alterations are initiated to resensitize the myofilament and restore systolic function.[47–49] Alternatively, HCM-associated mutations are typically characterized by increased calcium levels and reduced, prolonged calcium transients, despite progressive diastolic dysfunction with normal, or enhanced systolic function.[37,50–52] Thus, unlike DCM, these downstream disruptions suggest an uncoupling of the excitation-contraction pathway in HCM that potentiates disease pathogenesis (**Fig. 3**).

Many therapies implemented in the clinical management of heart failure have been targeted to restoring normal calcium homeostasis to improve diastolic and/or systolic function.[53,54] In a pilot trial

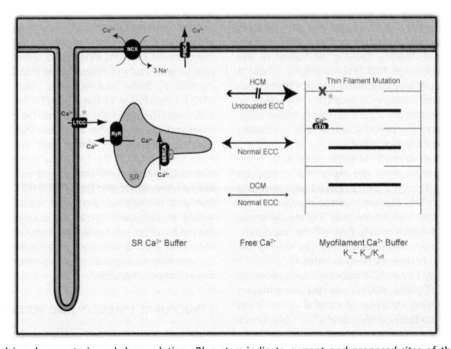

Fig. 3. Calcium homeostasis and dysregulation. *Blue stars* indicate current and proposed sites of therapeutic intervention for modulation of calcium homeostasis. NCX, Na-Ca, exchanger; PMCA, plasma membrane calcium ATP-ase; RyR, ryanodine receptor; SERCA, SR-bound calcium ATP-ase.

using diltiazem, an LTCC blocker, in a preclinical cohort of sarcomeric HCM, Ho and colleagues[53] described a reduction in progressive diastolic dysfunction and cardiac remodeling with treatment. Furthermore, after treatment cessation, progressive cardiac remodeling occurred, implicating diltiazem as an early intervention for HCM patients. Of note, the trial demonstrated early intervention for patients carrying *MYBPC3* mutations, whereas *MYH7* mutation carriers exhibited progressive cardiac remodeling and continued diastolic dysfunction throughout treatment.[53,55] The authors speculated a gene-specific response to diltiazem treatment, highlighting the necessity of defining the natural history of disease pathogenesis to implement efficacious interventions.

Therapeutics targeted to restoring calcium sensitivity of the myofilament have been proposed to be a more direct intervention in calcium homeostasis. To date, although small molecule calcium sensitizers have been successful in clinical trials at restoring cardiac function, the complexity of adverse effects make these therapies less than desirable for patients.[56] To improve these therapies, studies are ongoing to understand the precise mechanisms by which cTnC and the TF modulate calcium sensitivity. These advancements include additional small molecules (ie, EMD 57033) and the design of engineered cTnC variants, which have been shown to be a potential gene therapy option for modulating calcium sensitization.[57–59] Although the paradigm of calcium sensitivity offers insight into alterations in myofilament calcium handling, it is a steady-state measurement, thereby lacking resolution of the dynamic processes that govern affinity. Thus, it is imperative to investigate the kinetics of myofilament calcium handling, specifically the rates of calcium association (k_{on}) and dissociation (k_{off}), to understand the dynamic alterations mediating this divergent calcium affinity.

Myofilament calcium kinetics have long been overlooked because of the rapid rate of calcium exchange with cTnC as compared with the rate of relaxation.[60,61] Recent studies, however, have suggested that these rates may link the dynamic, myofilament-driven insults that initiate the downstream calcium dysregulation to the differential presentation of disease seen in patients.[11,60,62–65] For example, three HCM-causative mutations all found in cTnT (R92L, R92W, and R92Q) are known to have varying degrees of cardiac remodeling and risk of sudden cardiac death.[66–69] Myofibers independently expressing these mutations were shown to have nearly identical increases in calcium sensitivity of force generation[46,70] but differential downstream calcium dysregulation.[37,71]

Investigation into the dissociation kinetics revealed no change in the k_{off} for cTnT-R92Q TFs,[60] whereas cTnT-R92L and cTnT-R92W caused a significant decrease and increase in k_{off}, respectively.[11] These data suggest that the comparable increase in calcium affinity is likely the result of mutation-specific alterations in dynamic myofilament calcium handling.

Further investigation regarding the structural effects via MDS revealed mutation-specific repositioning of the N-terminus of cTnI, with respect to the calcium binding pocket that, in part, governed these changes in dissociation rate.[11] In parallel, a series of studies coupling *in silico*, *in vitro*, and *in vivo* approaches suggested that changes in calcium kinetics at the level of the TF and thus calcium homeostasis may also be regulated by an altered affinity of cTnI for actin and/or cTnC.[62,63,72] Although these studies were primarily focused on integrating the structural and functional responses of numerous phosphorylation events of cTnI, cardiomyopathy-associated mutations are known to propagate their effects to the critical cTnI-cTnC interface, as discussed previously. It follows that baseline structural insults that result in altered myofilament calcium sensitivity are likely intrinsically linked to the phosphorylation potential of the cTn core. Thus, these primary structural alterations may represent a therapeutic target that simultaneously ameliorates alterations in calcium handling and phosphorylation potential.

Although it is implausible to design a small molecule specific to each mutation that changes myofilament calcium kinetics, a subset of therapies targeted to restoration of the structural insults caused by these mutations (ie, repositioning of cTnI for restitution of the cTnI-cTnC and/or cTnI-actin equilibrium) may prove to be an efficient intervention. Furthermore, these therapies may also be applied to patients that are shown to have an intact ECC (ie, DCM) by stabilizing these molecular interactions that play a primary role in calcium sensitivity and thus regulation of contraction and relaxation. Continued research investigating atomic level alterations coupled to whole animal function will further the knowledge of how structure informs function, making the end goal of rationally designed, targeted small molecule therapeutics attainable.

STRUCTURAL STABILITY AND FLEXIBILITY

It has become increasingly clear that binary classifications of disease mechanism in cardiomyopathies (eg, hypercontractile vs hypocontractile and calcium sensitized vs desensitized discussed previously) may not be sufficient to describe the heterogeneity of disease presentation necessary for efficacious treatment. To address this, investigation into linking the primary structural insult, caused by single amino acid substitutions, to changes in the stability of the myofilament protein and/or its ability to interact with neighboring proteins within the cardiac sarcomere is ongoing. Indeed, the function of the myofilament depends on its innate ability to transmit seemingly small structural changes to distant portions of the complex via allosteric activation.[14] In this case, perturbations caused by mutations could alter the native stability of individual proteins or protein-protein interfaces at sites spatially distinct from the primary biophysical insult. The consequences of these "effects-at-a-distance" lead to initiation of pathogenic downstream signaling and ultimately the complexity observed in sarcomeric cardiomyopathies.

Mutations in the motor domain of myosin have long been postulated to disrupt the formation of strong cross-bridges.[73] Recent improvements in the ability to purify functional human β-myosin have led to significant advances in determining the structural insults caused by mutations.[74] For instance, the β-myosin mutations M531R (left ventricular noncompaction) and S532P (DCM) located in an actin-binding interface differentially perturb the local structure.[73] A second study showed that R453C (HCM) decreases the structural stability of the motor head throughout the cross-bridge cycle, suggesting an alteration in ATP binding and/or hydrolysis.[75] Thus, it is possible that via changes in structural stability of the motor domain, these mutations could be disrupting a communication pathway for actin binding-sites.[76] These examples highlight the importance of myofilament protein and protein-protein interface stability for the function of this highly evolved multisubunit machine.

Another example of these crucial structural stabilities and protein-protein interfaces is the complex association of the proteins of the regulatory TF, responsible for transmitting the calcium status of the myocyte to the sarcomere and muscle contraction. A more comprehensive review of the mechanism of contraction is presented elsewhere.[77,78] Briefly, at the onset of contraction calcium-induced calcium-release leads to cTnC binding calcium (described previously). Through a series of allosteric rearrangements in cTn, Tm shifts into the actin groove exposing the myosin binding sites on actin and allowing for strong cross-bridge formation and force generation.[79] Central to TF function is the "gatekeeper" Tm whose position is a dynamic equilibrium, moving

over the surface of actin between three states: (1) blocked, (2) closed, and (3) open.[78–80] Although the movement of Tm between these three states is tightly regulated, it must remain semiflexible to rapidly couple myocellular calcium status to force generation.[81,82]

Governing the interface between actin and Tm are many weak electrostatic interactions that are central to the function of Tm in regulating cross-bridge formation.[78,80,83] Tm, an α-helical coiled-coil dimer, has a surface charge that is largely negative with pockets of mostly acidic residues contributing to its binding to actin[84,85]; it spans actin forming a continuous, flexible filament that strengthens its interaction with actin via interdigitating N- and C-termini (**Fig. 4**). The head-to-tail association of subsequent dimers is crucial for the polymerization of Tm, its affinity for actin, and its cooperativity.[86–89] Further stabilizing this head-to-tail overlap is the α-helical component of the cTnT N-terminal domain resulting in a five-helix bundle at the overlap.[11,30,81,90–93] This arrangement allows for the flexibility and stability

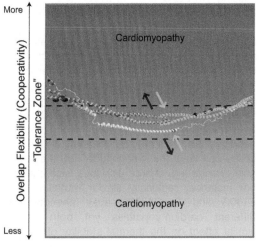

Fig. 4. Tm-overlap flexibility including the proposed "tolerance zone." The semiflexible Tm-overlap can vary within this zone (*dotted line*), becoming more (*purple*) or less (*blue*) flexible, outside of which is associated with disease. Overlaid on the gradient is the atomistic model generated from the publicly available average structure, by JR Exequiel Pineda, of the Tm N-terminus (*orange*), Tm C-terminus (*green*), and the N-terminal extension of cTnT (*yellow*).[11] The *arrows* represent decreased (*purple*) or increased (*blue*) interaction of the five-helix bundle that comprises the Tm-overlap. Included on the Tm and cTnT model are the sites of the discussed mutations (Tm-D175, E180, L185, E62, E40, E54, D84, D230, cTnT R92) with HCM in *red* and DCM in *dark blue*.

required to support the dynamic range of motion along actin necessary for the regulation of cross-bridge cycling.

Given the innate complexity of the system, it is not surprising that cardiomyopathy-associated mutations could locally alter the weak electrostatic interactions leading to propagation of structural effects to distant sites in cTn. In 2000 it was first posited that mutations altering the surface charge of Tm could be associated with DCM, whereby a charge reversal alters its electrostatic interactions with actin.[94] Furthermore, a large number of clinically relevant mutations exist near the Tm-overlap region, highlighting its functional significance. We and others have shown that such mutations on both Tm and cTnT propagate their structural effects altering Tm stability, Tm-overlap flexibility (cooperativity), and actin/cTnT affinity in a mutation-specific manner.[48,93,95–100] Notably, it was first postulated by Heller and colleagues[95] that alterations in thermal stability of the termini of Tm could translate to changes in Tm flexibility. In a study exploring the stability of Tm dimers containing the DCM-causing mutations Tm-E40K and Tm-E54K compared with the HCM causing Tm-E62Q and Tm-L185R it was shown that although the mutations did not affect the α-helical content of the Tm dimer, they did have a significant effect on the thermal denaturation (stability).[96] Similarly, we have shown that the DCM-causative Tm-D230N does not alter the α-helicity of Tm but leads to an increase in thermal stability of Tm-D230N dimers specifically at the C-terminus proximal to the mutation.[48] Strikingly the pathogenic outcome related to each mutation depends on the precise location within the coiled-coil and the "magnitude" of the amino acid change (eg, charge gain/loss, size change). For instance, regionally similar mutations Tm-E180G and Tm-D175N cause phenotypically different cardiomyopathies yet both had a similar effect on the thermal stability of Tm and increased local flexibility despite being in a Tn-binding pocket.[97,101,102] By contrast, the regionally distinct, mutations Tm-D84N and Tm-D230N result in the same charge loss and increase overall Tm stability and cause phenotypically different cardiomyopathies.[48,103–105] These changes in the absence of an altered secondary structure (helicity) suggest that the mutational effects could be propagating to the Tm-overlap, a highly sensitive functional domain, affecting its ability to regulate cross-bridge cycling. Furthermore, it suggests that the location of the mutation on Tm (coiled-coil position) and effects on regional stability of the individual proteins alone are not sufficient to predict pathogenicity.

Mutationally induced changes in Tm dimer interdigitation at the critical Tm-overlap could affect cooperativity, along its length, with adjacent Tm molecules and its ability to interact with actin and cTnT. Studies in reconstituted TFs have demonstrated that for some Tm mutations there is a change in the affinity of Tm for its neighboring proteins (cTnT and/or actin). For instance, with Tm-E180G and Tm-D175N it was shown that the affinity for actin was slightly reduced for Tm-D175N heterodimers (an effect that was much greater for Tm-D175N homodimers) with no apparent effect on the affinity for cTnT for either mutation.[100,101] Similarly, but in the opposite direction, mutations Tm-D84N and Tm-D230N demonstrated an increased affinity for actin.[103] These changes in actin affinity, although compelling, are likely not sufficient to explain the segregation of HCM and DCM given the complexity of the structural effects. In fact, studies comparing the HCM mutations Tm-E180G and Tm-E180V demonstrated that when bound to actin, Tm-E180G destabilized Tm suggesting a more flexible (less cooperative) Tm-overlap, whereas, in stark contrast, Tm-E180V strongly stabilized Tm suggesting a less flexible Tm-overlap.[106] Moreover, these affinity studies did not directly address the mutational effects on the complete Tm-overlap (containing actin, cTn, and Tm). To bridge this gap, we have recently demonstrated via in vitro experimentation coupled to computational modeling that the Tm-D230N mutation decreased the flexibility (increased cooperativity) of the full TF via compaction of the overlap region.[93] Furthermore, when the approach was extended to include the HCM-linked cTnT-R92L caused by its proximity to the overlap, a weaker overlap interaction (decreased stability) and more flexible (less cooperative) Tm was reported, in opposition to what was seen with DCM-linked Tm-D230N.[93] Lastly, recent studies on cardiomyopathy-associated mutations in a Tm-binding region of cTnT demonstrated altered binding affinity of cTnT for Tm whereby HCM mutations decreased affinity while DCM mutations increased affinity.[99] cTnT-R92L was shown to decrease affinity of cTnT for Tm correlating well with our previous findings. Of note, not all studied mutations fit this defined paradigm, indicating a regional specificity for the mutational effects.

Together these data suggest that mutations that give rise to cardiomyopathies can differentially affect both the stability of the affected protein and the flexibility of the critical overlap region independent of phenotypic outcome, leading to disease via distinct molecular mechanisms (see **Fig. 4**). It is likely that a complex interplay between stability and affinity governs pathogenicity dependent on the position of the mutation (eg, cTnT-binding domain, actin-binding domain) and the amino acid change. This complexity underscores the incomplete understanding of how single amino acid substitutions give rise to cardiomyopathies while simultaneously shedding light on the vast heterogeneity of disease presentation.

As with mutations that induce changes in calcium kinetics, it is likely implausible to generate small molecules to address the structural effects of each cardiomyopathy-causing mutation. However, understanding how a mutation alters the intramolecular and intermolecular allostery of affected proteins could lead to targeted therapies that correct specific sets of structural alterations. For instance, direct modulators of myosin function are in several phases of clinical trials.[107–109] Omecamtiv mecarbil, a cardiac myosin activator in testing for its efficacy in patients with systolic heart failure, has been shown to directly bind myosin S1 near the actin-binding domain favoring the strongly bound (open) force-generating state. Alternatively, mavacamten (MYK-461) has been shown to directly modulate contractility via decreasing enzymatic activity of myosin and the population of strongly bound cross-bridges in HCM.[108,109] Similarly, small molecules could be designed that target the TF with the goal of optimizing Tm cooperativity (via stabilization or destabilization of the overlap) toward a "tolerance zone" (see **Fig. 4**). Although work continues on understanding mutationally induced structural effects of the Tm-overlap, future studies will provide insight into the design of targeted molecules that act to ameliorate altered Tm flexibility at the earliest stages.

SUMMARY

This article focuses three "bins" that comprise sets of biophysical changes elicited by cardiomyopathy-linked mutations in the myofilament: (1) altered interaction of the cTnI-cTnC interface, (2) changes in calcium kinetics, and (3) altered protein stability and flexibility. The current binary paradigm of proposed mechanisms has proven to be inadequate to describe the heterogeneity of disease presentation. Although current therapies focus on symptom palliation, we and others have proposed that a more nuanced classification could lead to direct interventions based on the earliest dysregulation. Such early, targeted therapies could change the trajectory of disease progression in the preclinical cohort. Notably, the "bins" discussed here are a subset of this complexity and do not address other known

avenues including energetics, sarcomere assembly, and protein turnover. Continued research is necessary to address the complexity of cardiomyopathic progression and develop efficacious therapeutics.

REFERENCES

1. Geisterfer-Lowrance AA, Kass S, Tanigawa G, et al. A molecular basis for familial hypertrophic cardiomyopathy: a beta cardiac myosin heavy chain gene missense mutation. Cell 1990;62:999–1006.
2. Keren A, Syrris P, McKenna WJ. Hypertrophic cardiomyopathy: the genetic determinants of clinical disease expression. Nat Clin Pract Cardiovasc Med 2008;5:158.
3. McNally EM, Mestroni L. Dilated cardiomyopathy: genetic determinants and mechanisms. Circ Res 2017;121:731–48.
4. Braunwald E. Cardiomyopathies. Circ Res 2017; 121:711.
5. Hwang TJ, Lauffenburger JC, Franklin JM, et al. Temporal trends and factors associated with cardiovascular drug development, 1990 to 2012. JACC: Basic to Translational Science 2016;1:301.
6. Gigli M, Begay RL, Morea G, et al. A review of the giant protein titin in clinical molecular diagnostics of cardiomyopathies. Front Cardiovasc Med 2016; 3:21.
7. Gerull B. The rapidly evolving role of titin in cardiac physiology and cardiomyopathy. Can J Cardiol 2015;31:1351–9.
8. Golbus J, Puckelwartz M, Fahrenbach J, et al. Population-based variation in cardiomyopathy genes. Circ Cardiovasc Genet 2012;5:391–9.
9. Solaro R, Rarick H. Troponin and tropomyosin: proteins that switch on and tune in the activity of cardiac myofilaments. Circ Res 1998;83:471–80.
10. Zhang R, Zhao J, Mandveno A, et al. Cardiac troponin I phosphorylation increases the rate of cardiac muscle relaxation. Circ Res 1995;76: 1028–35.
11. Williams MR, Lehman SJ, Tardiff JC, et al. Atomic resolution probe for allostery in the regulatory thin filament. Proc Natl Acad Sci U S A 2016;113: 3257–62.
12. Rao V, Cheng Y, Lindert S, et al. PKA phosphorylation of cardiac troponin I modulates activation and relaxation kinetics of ventricular myofibrils. Biophys J 2014;107:1196–204.
13. Kentish JC, McCloskey DT, Layland J, et al. Phosphorylation of troponin I by protein kinase A accelerates relaxation and crossbridge cycle kinetics in mouse ventricular muscle. Circ Res 2001;88:1059–65.
14. Manning E, Tardiff J, Schwartz S. A model of calcium activation of the cardiac thin filament. Biochemistry 2011;50:7405–13.

15. Chandra M, Dong WJ, Pan BS, et al. Effects of protein kinase A phosphorylation on signaling between cardiac troponin I and the N-terminal domain of cardiac troponin C. Biochemistry 1997; 36:13305–11.

16. Hwang PM, Cai F, Pineda-Sanabria SE, et al. The cardiac-specific N-terminal region of troponin I positions the regulatory domain of troponin C. Proc Natl Acad Sci U S A 2014;111:14412–7.

17. Najafi A, Sequeira V, Kuster DW, et al. Beta-adrenergic receptor signalling and its functional consequences in the diseased heart. Eur J Clin Invest 2016;46:362–74.

18. Schumacher C, Becker H, Conrads R, et al. Hypertrophic cardiomyopathy: a desensitized cardiac beta-adrenergic system in the presence of normal plasma catecholamine concentrations. Naunyn Schmiedebergs Arch Pharmacol 1995; 351:398–407.

19. Choudhury L, Guzzetti S, Lefroy DC, et al. Myocardial beta adrenoceptors and left ventricular function in hypertrophic cardiomyopathy. Heart 1996; 75:50–4.

20. Cho MC, Rapacciuolo A, Koch WJ, et al. Defective beta-adrenergic receptor signaling precedes the development of dilated cardiomyopathy in transgenic mice with calsequestrin overexpression. J Biol Chem 1999;274:22251–6.

21. Spirito P, Maron BJ, Chiarella F, et al. Diastolic abnormalities in patients with hypertrophic cardiomyopathy: relation to magnitude of left ventricular hypertrophy. Circulation 1985;72:310–6.

22. Takeda S, Yamashita A, Maeda K, et al. Structure of the core domain of human cardiac troponin in the Ca2+-saturated form. Nature 2003;424:35–41.

23. Vinogradova MV, Stone DB, Malanina GG, et al. Ca2+-regulated structural changes in troponin. Proc Natl Acad Sci U S A 2005;102:5038–43.

24. Papadaki M, Marston SB. The importance of intrinsically disordered segments of cardiac troponin in modulating function by phosphorylation and disease-causing mutations. Front Physiol 2016;7:508.

25. Edes I, Kiss E, Kitada Y, et al. Effects of Levosimendan, a cardiotonic agent targeted to troponin C, on cardiac function and on phosphorylation and Ca2+ sensitivity of cardiac myofibrils and sarcoplasmic reticulum in guinea pig heart. Circ Res 1995;77:107–13.

26. Robertson IM, Baryshnikova OK, Li MX, et al. Defining the binding site of levosimendan and its analogues in a regulatory cardiac troponin C-troponin I complex. Biochemistry 2008;47: 7485–95.

27. Kasikcioglu HA, Cam N. A review of levosimendan in the treatment of heart failure. Vasc Health Risk Manag 2006;2:389–400.

28. Abbate A, Van Tassell BW. Levosimendan in advanced heart failure: where do we stand? J Cardiovasc Pharmacol 2017 [Epub ahead of print].

29. Mehta RH, Leimberger JD, van Diepen S, et al. Levosimendan in patients with left ventricular dysfunction undergoing cardiac surgery. N Engl J Med 2017;376:2032–42.

30. Palm T, Graboski S, Hitchcock-DeGregori S, et al. Disease-causing mutations in cardiac troponin T: identification of a critical tropomyosin-binding region. Biophys J 2001;81:2827–37.

31. Biesiadecki BJ, Kobayashi T, Walker JS, et al. The troponin C G159D mutation blunts myofilament desensitization induced by troponin I Ser23/24 phosphorylation. Circ Res 2007;100:1486–93.

32. Cheng Y, Regnier M. Cardiac troponin structure-function and the influence of hypertrophic cardiomyopathy associated mutations on modulation of contractility. Arch Biochem Biophys 2016;601: 11–21.

33. Dvornikov AV, Smolin N, Zhang M, et al. Restrictive cardiomyopathy troponin I R145W mutation does not perturb myofilament length-dependent activation in human cardiac sarcomeres. J Biol Chem 2016;291:21817–28.

34. Cheng Y, Rao V, Tu AY, et al. Troponin I mutations R146G and R21C alter cardiac troponin function, contractile properties, and modulation by protein kinase A (PKA)-mediated phosphorylation. J Biol Chem 2015;290:27749–66.

35. Wang Y, Pinto JR, Solis RS, et al. Generation and functional characterization of knock-in mice harboring the cardiac troponin I-R21C mutation associated with hypertrophic cardiomyopathy. J Biol Chem 2012;287:2156–67.

36. Dweck D, Sanchez-Gonzalez MA, Chang AN, et al. Long term ablation of protein kinase A (PKA)-mediated cardiac troponin I phosphorylation leads to excitation-contraction uncoupling and diastolic dysfunction in a knock-in mouse model of hypertrophic cardiomyopathy. J Biol Chem 2014;289: 23097–111.

37. Guinto P, Haim T, Dowell-Martino C, et al. Temporal and mutation-specific alterations in ca2+ homeostasis differentially determine the progression of ctnt-related cardiomyopathies in murine models. Am J Physiol Heart Circ Physiol 2009; 297:H614–26.

38. Papadaki M, Vikhorev PG, Marston SB, et al. Uncoupling of myofilament Ca2+ sensitivity from troponin I phosphorylation by mutations can be reversed by epigallocatechin-3-gallate. Cardiovasc Res 2015;108:99–110.

39. Eisner DA, Caldwell JL, Kistamás K, et al. Calcium and excitation-contraction coupling in the heart. Circ Res 2017;121:181.

40. Hasenfuss G, Meyer M, Schillinger W, et al. Calcium handling proteins in the failing human heart. Basic Res Cardiol 1997;92:87–93.

41. Meyer M, Schillinger W, Pieske B, et al. Alterations of sarcoplasmic reticulum proteins in failing human dilated cardiomyopathy. Circulation 1995;92:778–84.

42. Helms AS, Alvarado FJ, Yob J, et al. Genotype-dependent and -independent calcium signaling dysregulation in human hypertrophic cardiomyopathy. Circulation 2016;134:1738–48.

43. Coppini R, Ferrantini C, Yao L, et al. Late sodium current inhibition reverses electromechanical dysfunction in human hypertrophic cardiomyopathy: clinical perspective. Circulation 2013;127:575.

44. Pan S, Sommese RF, Sallam KI, et al. Establishing disease causality for a novel gene variant in familial dilated cardiomyopathy using a functional in-vitro assay of regulated thin filaments and human cardiac myosin. BMC Med Genet 2015;16:97.

45. Sommese RF, Nag S, Sutton S, et al. Effects of troponin T cardiomyopathy mutations on the calcium sensitivity of the regulated thin filament and the actomyosin cross-bridge kinetics of human beta-cardiac myosin. PLoS One 2013;8:e83403.

46. Chandra M, Tschirgi M, Tardiff J. Increase in tension-dependent ATP consumption induced by cardiac troponin T mutation. Am J Physiol Heart Circ Physiol 2005;289:H2112–9.

47. Ramratnam M, Salama G, Sharma RK, et al. Gene-targeted mice with the human troponin T R141W mutation develop dilated cardiomyopathy with calcium desensitization. PLoS One 2016;11: e0167681.

48. Lynn ML, Tal Grinspan L, Holeman TA, et al. The structural basis of alpha-tropomyosin linked (Asp230Asn) familial dilated cardiomyopathy. J Mol Cell Cardiol 2017;108:127–37.

49. Du C, Morimoto S, Nishii K, et al. Knock-in mouse model of dilated cardiomyopathy caused by troponin mutation. Circ Res 2007;101:185–94.

50. Knollmann BC, Kirchhof P, Sirenko SG, et al. Familial hypertrophic cardiomyopathy-linked mutant troponin T causes stress-induced ventricular tachycardia and Ca2+-dependent action potential remodeling. Circ Res 2003;92:428–36.

51. Lan F, Lee AS, Liang P, et al. Abnormal calcium handling properties underlie familial hypertrophic cardiomyopathy pathology in patient-specific induced pluripotent stem cells. Cell Stem Cell 2013;12:101–13.

52. Flenner F, Friedrich FW, Ungeheuer N, et al. Ranolazine antagonizes catecholamine-induced dysfunction in isolated cardiomyocytes, but lacks long-term therapeutic effects in vivo in a mouse model of hypertrophic cardiomyopathy. Cardiovasc Res 2016;109:90–102.

53. Ho CY, Lakdawala NK, Cirino AL, et al. Diltiazem treatment for pre-clinical hypertrophic cardiomyopathy sarcomere mutation carriers: a pilot randomized trial to modify disease expression. JACC Heart Fail 2015;3:180–8.

54. Greenberg B, Butler J, Felker GM, et al. Calcium upregulation by percutaneous administration of gene therapy in patients with cardiac disease (CUPID 2): a randomised, multinational, double-blind, placebo-controlled, phase 2b trial. Lancet 2016;387:1178–86.

55. Ho CY, Cirino AL, Lakdawala NK, et al. Evolution of hypertrophic cardiomyopathy in sarcomere mutation carriers. Heart 2016;102:1805–12.

56. Pollesello P, Papp Z, Papp JG. Calcium sensitizers: what have we learned over the last 25 years? Int J Cardiol 2016;203:543–8.

57. Liu B, Lee RS, Biesiadecki BJ, et al. Engineered troponin C constructs correct disease-related cardiac myofilament calcium sensitivity. J Biol Chem 2012;287:20027–36.

58. Shettigar V, Zhang B, Little SC, et al. Rationally engineered troponin C modulates in vivo cardiac function and performance in health and disease. Nat Commun 2016;7:10794.

59. White J, Lee JA, Shah N, et al. Differential effects of the optical isomers of EMD 53998 on contraction and cytoplasmic Ca2+ in isolated ferret cardiac muscle. Circ Res 1993;73:61–70.

60. Liu B, Tikunova SB, Kline KP, et al. Disease-related cardiac troponins alter thin filament Ca2+ association and dissociation rates. PLoS One 2012;7: e38259.

61. Davis JP, Tikunova SB. Ca(2+) exchange with troponin C and cardiac muscle dynamics. Cardiovasc Res 2008;77:619–26.

62. Salhi HE, Hassel NC, Siddiqui JK, et al. Myofilament calcium sensitivity: mechanistic insight into TnI Ser-23/24 and Ser-150 phosphorylation integration. Front Physiol 2016;7:567.

63. Siddiqui JK, Tikunova SB, Walton SD, et al. Myofilament calcium sensitivity: consequences of the effective concentration of troponin I. Front Physiol 2016;7:632.

64. Salhi HE, Walton SD, Hassel NC, et al. Cardiac troponin I tyrosine 26 phosphorylation decreases myofilament Ca2+ sensitivity and accelerates deactivation. J Mol Cell Cardiol 2014; 76:257–64.

65. Little SC, Biesiadecki BJ, Kilic A, et al. The rates of Ca2+ dissociation and cross-bridge detachment from ventricular myofibrils as reported by a fluorescent cardiac troponin C. J Biol Chem 2012;287: 27930–40.

66. Moolman JC, Corfield VA, Posen B, et al. Sudden death due to troponin T mutations. J Am Coll Cardiol 1997;29:549–55.

67. Forissier JF, Carrier L, Farza H, et al. Codon 102 of the cardiac troponin T gene is a putative hot spot for mutations in familial hypertrophic cardiomyopathy. Circulation 1996;94:3069–73.

68. Thierfelder L, Watkins H, MacRae C, et al. Alpha-tropomyosin and cardiac troponin T mutations cause familial hypertrophic cardiomyopathy: a disease of the sarcomere. Cell 1994;77:701–12.

69. Watkins H, McKenna WJ, Thierfelder L, et al. Mutations in the genes for cardiac troponin T and alpha-tropomyosin in hypertrophic cardiomyopathy. N Engl J Med 1995;332:1058–64.

70. Chandra M, Rundell VL, Tardiff JC, et al. Ca(2+) activation of myofilaments from transgenic mouse hearts expressing R92Q mutant cardiac troponin T. Am J Physiol Heart Circ Physiol 2001;280:H705–13.

71. Ferrantini C, Coppini R, Pioner JM, et al. Pathogenesis of hypertrophic cardiomyopathy is mutation rather than disease specific: a comparison of the cardiac troponin T E163R and R92Q mouse models. J Am Heart Assoc 2017;6 [pii: e005407].

72. Chung JH, Biesiadecki BJ, Ziolo MT, et al. Myofilament calcium sensitivity: role in regulation of in vivo cardiac contraction and relaxation. Front Physiol 2016;7:562.

73. Aksel T, Choe Yu E, Sutton S, et al. Ensemble force changes that result from human cardiac myosin mutations and a small-molecule effector. Cell Rep 2015;11:910–20.

74. Resnicow DI, Deacon JC, Warrick HM, et al. Functional diversity among a family of human skeletal muscle myosin motors. Proc Natl Acad Sci U S A 2010;107:1053–8.

75. Bloemink M, Deacon J, Langer S, et al. The hypertrophic cardiomyopathy myosin mutation R453C alters ATP binding and hydrolysis of human cardiac beta-myosin. J Biol Chem 2014;289:5158–67.

76. Nikolaeva OP, Orlov VN, Bobkov AA, et al. Differential scanning calorimetric study of myosin subfragment 1 with tryptic cleavage at the N-terminal region of the heavy chain. Eur J Biochem 2002;269:5678–88.

77. Batters C, Veigel C, Homsher E, et al. To understand muscle you must take it apart. Front Physiol 2014;5:90.

78. Gordon AM, Homsher E, Regnier M. Regulation of contraction in striated muscle. Physiol Rev 2000;80:853–924.

79. McKillop D, Geeves M. Regulation of the interaction between actin and myosin subfragment 1: evidence for three states of the thin filament. Biophys J 1993;65:693–701.

80. Gordon A, Regnier M, Homsher E. Skeletal and cardiac muscle contraction activation: tropomyosin "rocks and rolls". News Physiol Sci 2001;16:49–55.

81. Li XE, Orzechowski M, Lehman W, et al. Structure and flexibility of the tropomyosin overlap junction. Biochem Biophys Res Commun 2014;446:304–8.

82. Li X, Lehman W, Fischer S. The relationship between curvature, flexibility and persistence length in the tropomyosin coiled-coil. J Struct Biol 2010;170:313–8.

83. Holmes K, Lehman W. Gestalt-binding of tropomyosin to actin filaments. J Muscle Res Cell Motil 2008;29:213–9.

84. Barua B, Pamula M, Hitchcock-DeGregori S. Evolutionarily conserved surface residues constitute actin binding sites of tropomyosin. Proc Natl Acad Sci U S A 2011;108:10150–5.

85. Barua B, Fagnant PM, Winkelmann DA, et al. A periodic pattern of evolutionarily conserved basic and acidic residues constitutes the binding interface of actin-tropomyosin. J Biol Chem 2013;288:9602–9.

86. Cho YJ, Liu J, Hitchcock-DeGregori SE. The amino terminus of muscle tropomyosin is a major determinant for function. J Biol Chem 1990;265:538–45.

87. Brown JH, Kim KH, Jun G, et al. Deciphering the design of the tropomyosin molecule. Proc Natl Acad Sci U S A 2001;98:8496–501.

88. Phillips G Jr, Fillers J, Cohen C. Tropomyosin crystal structure and muscle regulation. J Mol Biol 1986;192:111–31.

89. Mak AS, Smillie LB. Non-polymerizable tropomyosin: preparation, some properties and F-actin binding. Biochem Biophys Res Commun 1981;101:208–14.

90. Greenfield NJ, Huang YJ, Swapna GV, et al. Solution NMR structure of the junction between tropomyosin molecules: implications for actin binding and regulation. J Mol Biol 2006;364:80–96.

91. Murakami K, Stewart M, Nozawa K, et al. Structural basis for tropomyosin overlap in thin (actin) filaments and the generation of a molecular swivel by troponin-T. Proc Natl Acad Sci U S A 2008;105:7200–5.

92. Frye J, Klenchin VA, Rayment I. Structure of the tropomyosin overlap complex from chicken smooth muscle: insight into the diversity of N-terminal recognition. Biochemistry 2010;49:4908–20.

93. McConnell M, Tal Grinspan L, Williams MR, et al. Clinically divergent mutation effects on the structure and function of the human cardiac tropomyosin overlap. Biochemistry 2017;56:3403–13.

94. Olson TM, Kishimoto NY, Whitby FG, et al. Mutations that alter the surface charge of alpha-tropomyosin are associated with dilated cardiomyopathy. J Mol Cell Cardiol 2001;33:723–32.

95. Heller M, Nili M, Homsher E, et al. Cardiomyopathic tropomyosin mutations that increase thin filament Ca2+ sensitivity and tropomyosin N-domain flexibility. J Biol Chem 2003;278:41742–8.

96. Chang AN, Greenfield NJ, Singh A, et al. Structural and protein interaction effects of hypertrophic and dilated cardiomyopathic mutations in alpha-tropomyosin. Front Physiol 2014;5:460.

97. Kremneva E, Boussouf S, Nikolaeva O, et al. Effects of two familial hypertrophic cardiomyopathy mutations in alpha-tropomyosin, Asp175Asn and Glu180Gly, on the thermal unfolding of actin-bound tropomyosin. Biophys J 2004;87:3922–33.

98. Loong CKP, Zhou H-X, Chase PB. Familial hypertrophic cardiomyopathy related E180G mutation increases flexibility of human cardiac α-tropomyosin. FEBS Lett 2012;586:3503–7.

99. Gangadharan B, Sunitha MS, Mukherjee S, et al. Molecular mechanisms and structural features of cardiomyopathy-causing troponin T mutants in the tropomyosin overlap region. Proc Natl Acad Sci U S A 2017;114:11115–20.

100. Janco M, Kalyva A, Scellini B, et al. α-tropomyosin with a D175N or E180G mutation in only one chain differs from tropomyosin with mutations in both chains. Biochemistry 2012;51:9880–90.

101. Golitsina N, An Y, Greenfield NJ, et al. Effects of two familial hypertrophic cardiomyopathy-causing mutations on α-tropomyosin structure and function. Biochemistry 1997;36:4637–42.

102. White SP, Cohen C, Phillips GN Jr. Structure of co-crystals of tropomyosin and troponin. Nature 1987; 325:826.

103. Gupte TM, Haque F, Gangadharan B, et al. Mechanistic heterogeneity in contractile properties of alpha-tropomyosin (TPM1) mutants associated with inherited cardiomyopathies. J Biol Chem 2015;290:7003–15.

104. van de Meerakker JB, Christiaans I, Barnett P, et al. A novel alpha-tropomyosin mutation associates with dilated and non-compaction cardiomyopathy and diminishes actin binding. Biochim Biophys Acta 2013;1833:833–9.

105. Lakdawala N, Dellefave L, Redwood C, et al. Familial dilated cardiomyopathy caused by an alpha-tropomyosin mutation: the distinctive natural history of sarcomeric dilated cardiomyopathy. J Am Coll Cardiol 2010;55:320–9.

106. Matyushenko AM, Shchepkin DV, Kopylova GV, et al. Structural and functional effects of cardiomyopathy-causing mutations in the troponin T-binding region of cardiac tropomyosin. Biochemistry 2017;56:250–9.

107. Hwang PM, Sykes BD. Targeting the sarcomere to correct muscle function. Nat Rev Drug Discov 2015;14:313–28.

108. Green EM, Wakimoto H, Anderson RL, et al. A small-molecule inhibitor of sarcomere contractility suppresses hypertrophic cardiomyopathy in mice. Science 2016;351:617–21.

109. Kawas RF, Anderson RL, Ingle SRB, et al. A small-molecule modulator of cardiac myosin acts on multiple stages of the myosin chemomechanical cycle. J Biol Chem 2017;292: 16571–7.

Clinical and Molecular Aspects of Cardiomyopathies
Emerging Therapies and Clinical Trials

Niccolò Maurizi, MD[a],*, Enrico Ammirati, MD, PhD[b],
Raffaele Coppini, MD, PhD[c], Amelia Morrone, PhD[d],
Iacopo Olivotto, MD[a]

KEYWORDS

- Rare cardiac diseases • New therapies • Precision medicine • Genetics • Cardiomyopathies
- Clinical trials

KEY POINTS

- Cardiomyopathies are diseases of the myocardium, often genetically determined, associated with heterogeneous phenotypes and clinical manifestations.
- Despite significant progress in the understanding of these conditions, available treatments mostly target late complications, while approaches that promise to interfere with the primary mechanisms and natural history are just beginning to surface.
- The present review focuses on novel pharmacologic approaches to genetic cardiomyopathies, with a view to future developments and potential clinical implications.

Cardiomyopathies are diseases of the myocardium associated with heterogeneous morphofunctional phenotypes and clinical manifestations, frequently due to a genetic cause.[1] The last 2 decades have witnessed significant progress in the treatment of patients with cardiomyopathies, resulting in decreasing rates of mortality and morbidity.[2] However, available treatments largely target downstream complications, whereas approaches that promise to truly interfere with primary molecular mechanisms and change the natural history of myocardial disease are just beginning to surface.[3] Tailored pharmacologic therapies for cardiomyopathies remain an unmet

need and a research priority.[4] In recent years, the establishment of centers of excellence and large international registries has allowed the recruitment of sizable patient cohorts,[5] whereas advances in cardiac imaging and genetic testing, deeper understanding of the molecular targets, and growing involvement by the pharmaceutical industry have led to a rapid increase in the number of dedicated trials (**Fig. 1**, **Table 1**). Nevertheless, formidable challenges remain: even the most prevalent cardiomyopathies are relatively uncommon compared with "classic" cardiac diseases, and others are undeniably rare. Furthermore, clinical presentation and outcome are heterogeneous;

Disclosures: I. Olivotto has received research grants from Gilead, Menarini International, Sanofi Genzyme, Shire, Amicus, and Myokardia.
a Cardiomyopathy Unit, Careggi University Hospital, Florence, Italy; b "De Gasperis" Cardio Center and Transplant Center, ASST Grande Ospedale Metropolitano Niguarda, Milan, Italy; c Department NeuroFarBa, University of Florence, Florence, Italy; d Paediatric Neurology Unit and Laboratories, Neuroscience Department, Meyer Children's Hospital, Florence, Italy
* Corresponding author. Cardiomyopathy Unit, Careggi University Hospital, Viale Pieraccini 17, Florence 50132, Italy.
E-mail address: niccolo.maurizi@gmail.com

Heart Failure Clin 14 (2018) 161–178
https://doi.org/10.1016/j.hfc.2018.01.001

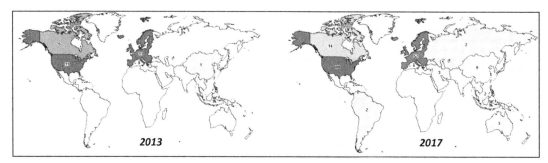

Fig. 1. Number of HCM registered trials across the world in 2013 and 2017. (*From* https://clinicaltrials.gov/ct2/results/map?term=hypertrophic+cardiomyopathy&map=.)

"hard" event rates are low, and resources are limited.[6] Most existing trials have targeted only specific subsets of patients and have necessarily used surrogate endpoints such as indexes of functional capacity or changes in left ventricular (LV) mass, fibrosis, and outflow gradients.[5] None was ever powered to assess the impact of therapeutic interventions on clinical course and outcome. Thus, even potentially effective drugs might fail to show their benefit due to inadequate endpoints, sample size, and time span of clinical experimentation. Consequently, the need for novel, specific trial design is emerging for these slowly progressive, chronic conditions largely affecting young individuals.[7]

The present review focuses on novel pharmacologic approaches to genetic cardiomyopathies, with a view to future developments and potential clinical implications. There are different levels of interventions that are being pursued, ranging from the most accessible, but less satisfactory, relief of symptoms, to more ambitious but still embryonic approaches attempting to prevent or reverse disease phenotypes (**Fig. 2**). Because it is not feasible to address the multitude of conditions in which research is ongoing, the authors have limited their focus to the principal paradigms, in order to illustrate the state of the art in the field.

EMERGING STRATEGIES FOR HYPERTROPHIC CARDIOMYOPATHY

Hypertrophic cardiomyopathy (HCM) is a common genetic disorder characterized by cardiac hypertrophy not explained by abnormal loading conditions, largely caused by genes coding for proteins of the sarcomere.[8] HCM has a 1:500 prevalence in the general population and represents a frequent cause of sudden cardiac death in the young, although the absolute incidence of events is rare.[2] Pharmacologic therapy plays a very important role in restoring quality of life and reducing risk of complications. Plausible options

under investigation include the repurposing of well-known drugs, such as diltiazem or ranolazine, as well as development of novel agents targeting disease-specific abnormalities.[9] At the clinical level, current pharmacologic research focuses on 2 different approaches: modifiers of overt clinical HCM phenotypes and prevention of phenotype development in genotype positive "healthy" individuals.

Overt Hypertrophic Cardiomyopathy

One of the most intriguing hypotheses explaining HCM pathogenesis focuses on excess sarcomere activation and energy expenditure as the primary defect in HCM. Sarcomere mutations causing HCM are generally gain of function, producing overactivation of the contractile apparatus and profound metabolic changes ultimately leading to energy depletion and triggering of fibrosis.[10] A small-molecule allosteric myosin inhibitor, mavacamten (MYK-461; Myokardia, San Francisco, CA, USA), has recently been developed to restore physiologic contractile and energetic balance in HCM hearts by decreasing adenosine triphosphatase activity of the cardiac myosin heavy chain.[11] In an HCM mouse model, mavacamten effectively prevented development of LVH, myocyte disarray, and fibrosis and downregulated both hypertrophic and profibrotic gene expression[11] (**Fig. 3**). Phenotype reversal was observed in early stages, but not in older mice.[11] Human studies are now underway, and a phase 2 study has recently been completed to evaluate the efficacy, safety, and tolerability of mavacamten in subjects with symptomatic HCM and left ventricular outflow tract (LVOT) obstruction (NCT02842242); a large phase 2/3 study is due to start in 2018.

A previous attempt to reduce the energetic cost of the HCM myocardium and improve its efficiency was performed with perhexiline, a metabolic modulator that inhibits free fatty acid metabolism and enhances carbohydrate utilization by

Table 1
Ongoing or recently completed clinical trials addressing patients with cardiomyopathies associated with specific gene mutations

Disease	Drug	Patients	Molecular Target/Effects in Preclinical Studies	Clinical Study	Number of Patients	Expected Results	Identifier	Status
HCM	Diltiazem	Sarcomere mutation carriers without clinically evident HCM	Reduced Ca entry into the cytosol of CMs, causing ↓ [Ca]i, therefore prevention of hypertrophy and LV dysfunction	Randomized, placebo-controlled, double-blind clinical trial randomly assigned to diltiazem 360 mg/d (or 5 mg/kg/d) or placebo for 25 mo	38 participants, 18 in the diltiazem group and 20 controls aged 5–39 y old	Exploratory analysis of phenotype development prevention among mutation carriers	NCT00319982	Completed
	Losartan/Valsartan	Sarcomere mutation carriers without clinically evident HCM	AT1-receptor blockers on CMs and myocardial FBs	Randomized, placebo-controlled, double-blind clinical trial randomly assigned to valsartan 80–320 mg daily (depending on age and weight) or placebo	150 patients aged 8–45 y old	Stability/attenuation of progression in metrics of LV and left atrial size, LV systolic/diastolic function, metabolic exercise testing, proBNP, collagen markers	NCT01912534	Enrolling
	Ranolazine	Clinically diagnosed HCM in NYHA class II-III and peak Vo2 <75% of predicted	Late Na current of CMs, based on reduction of cellular arrhythmogenesis, improved diastolic function	Phase 2 study with nonobstructive HCM randomly assigned to placebo (n = 40) or ranolazine 1000 mg bid (n = 40) for 5 mo	80 adult patients aged 18–65 y old	Improvement in functional capacity, diastolic function, proBNP, arrhythmic profile, and quality of life from enrollment	EUDRA-CT: 2011-004507-20	Completed

(continued on next page)

Table 1
(continued)

Disease	Drug	Patients	Molecular Target/Effects in Preclinical Studies	Clinical Study	Number of Patients	Expected Results	Identifier	Status
	Perhexiline	Clinically diagnosed nonobstructive HCM and peak Vo_2 <75% of predicted	By shifting substrate to more efficient carbohydrate metabolism, increase exercise capacity by improving cardiac energetics and LV relaxation	Phase 2 study randomized, double-blind, placebo-controlled of 3–6 mo; during entire duration received either perhexiline 100 mg (n = 24) or placebo (n = 22)	46 adult patients aged 18–80 y old	Reduction in myocardial ratio of phosphocreatine to ATP, improvement in LV diastolic filling, peak Vo_2, symptoms, quality of life, and serum metabolites	NCT00500552	Completed
	Eleclazine	Clinically diagnosed HCM with LVOT obstruction in NYHA class II-III and peak Vo_2 <75% of predicted	Late Na current of CMs, based on reduction of cellular arrhythmogenesis, improved diastolic function	Phase 2 study with obstructive HCM patients randomly assigned to placebo (n = 75) or eleclazine (n = 75) for 24 wk	150 adult patients aged 18–65 y old	Improvement in functional capacity, diastolic function, proBNP, arrhythmic profile, reduction of LVOT gradient, and quality of life from enrollment	NCT02291237	Interrupted
	Mavacampten	Clinically diagnosed nonobstructive HCM and NYHA >I	Myosing head inhibition promotes better energetic and gradient drops	Open-label phase 2 study single group assignment	21 adult patients aged 18–70 y old	Change in postexercise peak LVOT gradient from baseline to week 1	NCT02842242	Completed

	Drug	Indication	Mechanism	Study	Patients	Outcome	Trial / Status
Dilated cardio myopathies	ARRY-371797	DCM due to LMNA gene mutation	Oral p38 inhibitor	Phase 2: safety study sponsored by Array BioPharma, USA	12 patients 24 mo follow-up	Drug safety and efficacy terms of 6-min walking time, LV and RV function, quality of life	NCT02351856 Recruiting
	Perindopril	Genotype-positive phenotype-negative DCM	Known molecular targets of ACEi	PRECARDIA, multicenter European double-blind randomized trial (perindopril vs placebo 1:1 ratio) sponsored by INSERM, France	200 participants with carriers of mutations identified in the family as associated with a DCM (age 19–59 y)	ACEi may delay or prevent the occurrence of DCM (LVEF <45%) in these subjects (preclinical stage) at 36 mo	NCT01583114 Completed
	Eteplirsen	DMD patients that are amenable to skipping exon 51	Administration of 2'-O-methyl RNA phosphorothioate AON targeting exon 51 of the gene showed restoration of dystrophin in the injected muscle	An open-label, multicenter, study with a concurrent untreated control arm to evaluate the efficacy and safety of eteplirsen in DMD	160 patients IV injection of eteplirsen 30 mg/kg for 96 wk	Improvement in functional capacity as measured by 6-min walking test; muscle biopsy at enrollment and last visit	NCT02255552 Active, not recruiting

(continued on next page)

Table 1
(continued)

Disease	Drug	Patients	Molecular Target/Effects in Preclinical Studies	Clinical Study	Number of Patients	Expected Results	Identifier	Status
	Allogeneic cardiosphere-derived cells (CAP-1002)	DMD cardio-myopathy	CAP-1002 has a potent immuno-modulatory activity that alters the immune system's activity to encourage cellular regeneration	Randomized open-label usual care controlled multicenter study the safety and preliminary efficacy of intracoronary CAP-1002	25 male patients with Duchenne cardiomyopathy with LV scar involving at least 4 cardiac segments, ejection fraction $\geq$35%	Safety and phenotype development prevention as assessed with MRI and serum biomarkers	NCT02485938	Recruiting
	Eplerenone	Subclinical DMD cardio-myopathy	In mouse model eplerenone prevents Duchenne cardiomyopathy development	Randomized parallel control trial with participants allocated to eplerenone 25 mg tablet or placebo	42 patients aged more than 7 mo	12-mo change in myocardial strain	NCT01521546	Completed
Metabolic cardio myopathies	Migalastat	Fabry cardio-myopathy	Promotion of correct protein folding and functioning	Randomized placebo controlled trial with migalastat 150 mg or placebo	67 patients with amenable FD mutation	Change in lyso-GB3, creatinine, and LV mass	NCT01218659	Completed

cardiomyocytes.[12] In a randomized, double-blind placebo-controlled trial, perhexiline was able to improve myocardial phosphocreatine to adenosine triphosphate ratio, resulting in improved diastolic function and exercise capacity in HCM patients.[13] However, concerns exist regarding the safety profile of the drug, following reports of hepatotoxicity in predisposed individuals, and the drug requires long-term monitoring of plasma levels.[13] A confirmatory trial assessing the efficacy of perhexiline in HCM was designed but recently withdrawn (https://clinicaltrials.gov/ct2/show/NCT02431221).

HCM is associated with complex electrophysiological remodeling at the cellular level. In a study from the authors' group, the late sodium current (INaL) was markedly overexpressed in isolated human HCM cardiomyocytes, causing intracellular calcium overload and enhanced arrhythmic propensity[14] (**Fig. 4**). Selective INaL inhibition by ranolazine substantially improved these abnormalities in vitro.[14] A multicenter double-blind, placebo-controlled pilot study was performed to test the efficacy of ranolazine on exercise capacity in symptomatic patients with nonobstructive HCM. Overall, ranolazine showed no effect on functional capacity, diastolic function, and quality of life, despite improving plasma ProBNP levels and reducing the 24-hour burden of ventricular ectopies.[15] Almost one-third of patients in the ranolazine groups appeared to respond to treatment, with increases in peak Vo_2 >2 mL/kg/m compared with baseline; however, individual variability was considerable, and most patients did not show any benefit. This trend is in line with recent observations in transgenic HCM mice, suggesting marked genetic variability in the degree of INaL overexpression (which appeared to be mutation specific) and consequently in the individual response to INaL blockade.[16] Recently, eleclazine (GS-6615; Gilead Sciences, Foster City, CA, USA), a new more potent and selective inhibitor of INaL has been developed. In order to test whether, compared with placebo, eleclazine improved exercise capacity in subjects with symptomatic HCM, the LIBERTY-HCM trial (GS-US-361-1157) was designed.[5,17] It was the largest trial yet performed in HCM, recruiting 172 patients from more than 40 centers in Europe and the United States. The first study subject was screened in February 2015. Unfortunately, in November 2016, because of a higher incidence rate of implantable cardioverter-defibrillator (ICD) shocks in eleclazine-treated subjects in a parallel phase 2 study enrolling subjects with ventricular tachycardia/ventricular fibrillation and

ICDs (GS-US-356-0101, TEMPO), Liberty-HCM was discontinued and the eleclazine development program was interrupted.

Phenotype Prevention

Recent developments in genome-editing techniques and their successful application in animal models have provided an option for correcting human germline mutations. Three main experimental approaches are being been tested in HCM, including adeno-associated virus (AAV9)-Mybpc3 transfection in mice, allele-specific silencing via RNA interference, and CRISPR-Cas9 editing.[18–20] In 2017, Ma and coworkers[20] by using CRISPR-Cas9 were able to correct a heterozygous MYBPC3 mutation in human preimplantation embryos, avoiding mosaicism in cleaving embryos and achieving a high yield of homozygous human embryos carrying the wild-type MYBPC3 gene without evidence of off-target mutations. Although the applicability of such approach to other HCM-causing defects and its reproducibility in clinical practice are still unresolved, these important findings support the potential for correction of heritable mutations in human embryos.[20]

Several pharmacologic attempts have been made to prevent development of left ventricular hypertrophy (LVH) in phenotype-negative individuals carrying HCM-causing mutations, by addressing the principal downstream molecular abnormalities triggered by the genetic defect.[9,21] Based on the observation that such variants trigger dysregulation of intracellular calcium handling, preclinical administration of diltiazem has been successfully used in a mouse HCM model to correct early LV remodeling.[9] In a pilot, double-blind trial enrolling 38 young sarcomere mutation carriers, therapy with diltiazem 360 mg per day for a median of 25 months attenuated the longitudinal decrease in LV cavity size observed in the placebo group. The improvements were lost within a year after treatment was stopped, suggesting a significant impact of the drug.[21]

A similar approach aims to counter the activation of tumor growth factor-β, occurring early in HCM pathogenesis, by angiotensin II type 1 receptor blockers (ARBs).[4] With this purpose, the ongoing VANISH randomized trial has enrolled preclinical HCM mutation carriers to evaluate the efficacy of disease-modifying therapy with valsartan for prevention of phenotype development.[22] In patients with fully developed HCM, however, earlier hopes that ARBs might improve cardiac phenotype[23] were not confirmed in a larger, randomized trial based on cardiac MRI, which failed

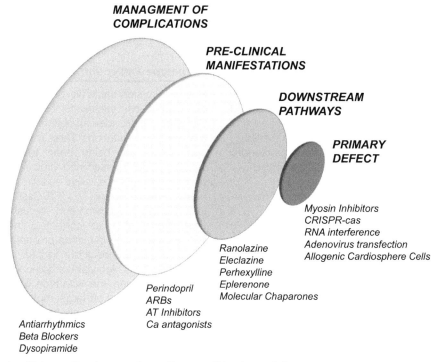

Fig. 2. Levels of intervention for genetic cardiomyopathies: toward the core.

to show any effect of losartan on LVH and fibrosis at 12 months.[24]

Long-term treatment with N-acetylcysteine (NAC), a precursor to the most abundant intracellular nonprotein thiol pool against oxidative stress, reversed cardiac hypertrophy and interstitial fibrosis in a transgenic rabbit HCM model, suggesting potential beneficial effects in reversal of cardiac phenotype.[25] However, no human data are available with this molecule. In the same animal model, the administration of atorvastatin prevented the development of LVH over a 1-year period. As for NAC, this effect was attributed to a reduction in oxidative stress.[26] A small pilot study with atorvastatin, however, failed to show any clinical or instrumental benefit in HCM patients.[27]

NOVEL APPROACHES TO DILATED CARDIOMYOPATHY OF GENETIC CAUSE

Dilated cardiomyopathy (DCM) is characterized by ventricular chamber enlargement, systolic dysfunction, and LV mass increase with normal wall thickness and affects relatively young individuals, accounting for 40% to 50% of heart transplantations.[1] In a substantial proportion of DCM patients, the disease has a genetic cause.[28]

Treatment of genetic DCM has classically followed the tenets of systolic heart failure (HF) management, benefiting hugely from the pharmacologic armamentarium developed in the last 3 decades (culminating in the recent introduction of sacubitril/valsartan), as well as CRT, whereas the role of the ICD is more controversial in this setting.[29,30] Further advances, however, will require leaving behind the classic one-fits-all approach in favor of a tailored line of attack, particularly in the case of genetic disease.[31]

Genetics can be useful in the management of DCM patients in various ways. First, it can identify patients with molecular targets specifically related to biophysical consequences of their mutations, allowing the development of selective agents. Second, it can identify subsets of patients gaining greater benefit from approved drugs or devices. Third, as for HCM, it allows early identification of genotype-positive phenotype-negative individuals who can be preemptively treated in the attempt to prevent or delay the onset of disease.[31]

The spectrum of genes, molecules, and cellular pathways involved in DCM is considerably more complex than in HCM. Although a sarcomeric cause is described, it is uncommon, accounting only for 7% to 10% of DCM. More often, mutations affect genes coding for proteins involved in force transmission, such as *TTN* encoding for titin.[32,33] Titin truncation defects (*TTNtv*) are the most common single cause of genetic DCM, accounting for 20% to 30% of cases. Related to these are mutations in RBM20, a chaperon protein encoding the

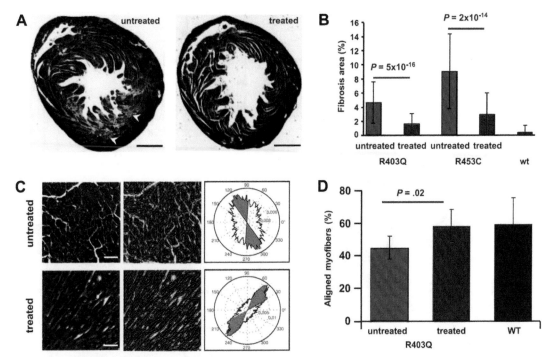

Fig. 3. MYK-461 reduces the development of myocardial disarray and fibrosis in mouse models of HCM. (*A*) Sections from untreated (*left*) and MYK-461-treated (*right*) 30-week-old R403Q mice stained with Masson's trichrome (*arrowheads*, fibrotic areas). Scale bars, 1 mm. (*B*) Reduction in fibrosis area with MYK-461 treatment assessed in more than 8 sections per mouse for R403Q and R453C HCM mice (n = 5–6 animals per group). (*C*) Representative regions of interest for analysis of cell orientation fromR403Q mouse heart sections. Regions are shown (*left*) stained with Masson's trichrome (scale bars, 50 μM), (*middle*) with local gradient vectors illustrating cell orientations for analysis, and (*right*) as rose plots of the distribution of myofibril orientation angles (*blue line*; myofibrils oriented within 20° of the mean are shaded in red). (*D*) Percentage of aligned myofibers in wild-type (WT) and R403Q mice with and without MYK-461 treatment (n = 6 animals per condition). (*From* Green EM, Wakimoto H, Anderson RL. A small-molecule inhibitor of sarcomere contractility suppresses hypertrophic cardiomyopathy in mice. Science 2016;351(6273):619; with permission.)

ribonucleic acid binding motif 20, which lead to titin splicing.[34] Other biological pathways involve disorder in calcium homeostasis, epitomized by phospholamban mutations (*PLN* gene)[34] and abnormalities in the transmembrane cardiac voltage-gated sodium channel encoded by *SCN5A* gene, whose defects cause a DCM phenotype associated with marked arrhythmic propensity.[35] Last but not least, mutations in the *LMNA* gene, encoding lamin A/C, affect the structural organization and stability of the nuclear envelope. *LMNA* gene variants are found in approximately 6% of DCM cases, characterized by progressive LV dysfunction associated with severe conduction disease, atrial fibrillation, and risk of sudden cardiac death, warranting early consideration for an ICD even at early stages of LV dysfunction.[36,37] In the retrospective study by Meune and colleagues,[37] 42% of patients with progressive conduction block received an appropriate ICD intervention after a mean follow-up of 34 months,

despite a mean left ventricular ejection fraction (LVEF) of 58%. Thus, primary prevention of sudden cardiac death in Lamin A/C DCM represents a very good example of genetically driven management of DCM. Several specific pharmacologic approaches are also being developed for this condition.[38] Cardiac mitogen-activated protein kinases (MAPKs) and protein kinase B (AKT)/ mammalian target of rapamycin (mTOR) signaling pathways are overactivated in Lamin A/C hearts. Thus, several MAPK and AKT/mTOR pathway inhibitors are under scrutiny, including MEK1/2 inhibitors, c-Jun N-terminal kinase inhibitors, and p38α inhibitors. The latter is under investigation in a small phase 2 study trial of Lamin A/C DCM (NCT02351856).[39] Other approaches include restoration of cellular autophagy by temsirolimus and an antisense oligonucleotide strategy (limited to missense mutations in exon 11) aimed at reducing prelamin A and tipping the balance of splicing toward lamin C.[38]

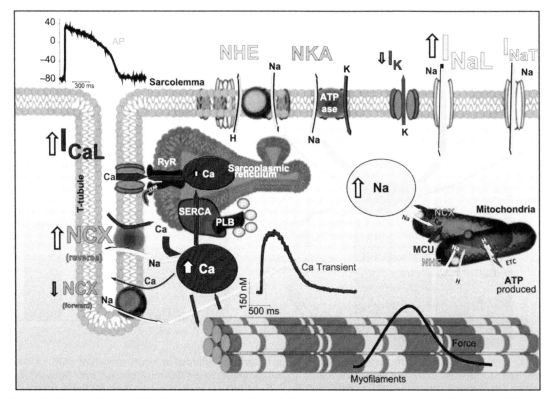

Fig. 4. Na homeostasis in HCM. Cartoon showing the cellular and molecular determinants of abnormal Naþ homeostasis in cardiac cells from HCM patients and their role in determining the dysfunction of Ca2þ handling and contraction. White thick arrows mark the changes occurring in HCM with respect to control cardiomyocytes. The thickness of yellow and blue arrows has been changed to match the relative changes of Naþ and Ca2þ fluxes in HCM versus control cells. AP, Action Potential; ATP, Adenosine Tri Phosphate; Ca L, Calcium L channel; NaL, Na L Channel; NCX, Sodium Calcium Exchanger; NHE, Sodium Hydrogen Antiporter; NKA, Sodium Potassium ATPase0. (*Adapted from* Coppini R, Ferrantini C, Yao L. Late sodium current inhibition reverses electro-mechanical dysfunction in human hypertrophic cardiomyopathy. Circulation 2013;127(5):582.)

Duchenne Muscular Dystrophy

X-linked Duchenne muscular dystrophy (DMD), the most common childhood muscle disease, is caused by an absence of the dystrophin protein, encoded by the DMD gene, in skeletal muscle fibers[40] and represents an important cause of juvenile DCM. The disease is characterized by progressive skeletal and cardiac muscle degeneration, loss of ambulation, and premature death caused by cardiac and/or respiratory failure.[40,41] The *DMD* gene, composed of 79 constitutive exons, is one of the largest human genes.[40] More than 7000 *DMD* gene mutations have been reported (https://www. qiagenbioinformatics.com/products/human-gene-mutation-database/; https://databases.lovd.nl/ shared/genes/DMD; https://www.ncbi.nlm.nih.gov/ clinvar/?term=DMD%5Bgene%5D). Of these, 80% are intragenic rearrangements with deletions or duplications of one exon (such as exon 52) or more exons (exons 42–44). Single or multiple exon deletions leading to a frameshift of the DMD gene

open reading frame (ORF) lead to a DMD phenotype. Deletions and/or insertions that do not disrupt the ORF lead to the milder Becker phenotype.[42,43] Restoration of ORF can lead to the synthesis of a mutated but functional dystrophin protein even if it differs in quality, quantity, and length from the wild-type protein.

Restoration of dystrophin expression by innovative therapeutic approaches has been one of the main research goals in the field in the last 2 decades.[42,44] These strategies can be categorized as genetic or molecular therapies.[45] Genetic therapies include all kinds of manipulation that introduce genetic material, such as a functioning gene or a recombinant DNA gene copy, in the patient's cells to correct total or partial deletion or inactive/altered transcription or translation (**Table 2**). Molecular therapy refers to the use of small or large molecules (oligonucleotide, chaperones, or proteins/enzymes) that interact with the patient's endogenous genetic material, transcription, or translation, restoring the endogenous

Table 2
Primary genetic defects and proposed therapeutic approaches

Type of Primary Gene Defect	Transcriptional Effect	Potential Treatment Approach
Gene rearrangement	Total absence or aberrant protein	Gene therapy, enzyme replacement therapy, or exon skipping therapy
RNA defects due to splicing defects or deep intronic mutations	RNA aberrant transcripts with or without the synthesis of aberrant proteins	Gene therapy, enzyme replacement therapy, or exon skipping therapy
Single nucleotide change	Amino acid changes leading to premature stop codons	Stop codon read-through therapy
Posttranscriptional modifications	Late-onset phenotype and residual enzyme/protein	Pharmacologic chaperone therapy

cellular mechanism leading to the production of the patient's own product. A variety of approaches that include genetic manipulation have been attempted, such as exon skipping,[41] read-through therapy,[45] gene therapy with viral vectors, and cell therapy.[46] Recently, CRISPR-Cas9 technology has been used to edit the patient's genome.[47]

Targeted exon-skipping therapy, the most promising approach to date, based on the use of antisense oligonucleotides (AONs),[48] aims to correct the disrupted reading frame of the dystrophin-encoding gene.[41] AONs are synthesized to bind to complementary sequences of the target pre–messenger RNA (mRNA) used for splicing modulation and induce a corrective in frame exon skipping that restores the synthesis of a partly functional protein. By so doing, exon skipping therapy for DMD results in the conversion of severe DMD to the milder Becker muscular dystrophy.[49]

The administration of 2'-O-methyl RNA phosphorothioate AON and of morpholino AON, targeting exon 51 of the gene that accounts for ≈13% of DMD mutations, showed promising restoration of dystrophin in the injected muscle.[50] Two AONs, drisapersen and eteplirsen, have entered human experimentation. Initial phase 1 and 2 trials for both eteplirsen and drisapersen succeeded in restoring dystrophin expression, but did not show benefit in the primary endpoint, the 6-minute walk test.[41,51] In the phase 3 PROMOVI trial, eteplirsen significantly increased dystrophin levels from baseline in muscle tissues of 12 patients after 48 weeks of treatment and reduced the rate of ambulation and pulmonary function decline.[52,53] In September 2016, the US Food and Drug Administration granted accelerated approval for eteplirsen in DMD patients with amenable genetic variants in exon 51.[53]

Gene Transfer Approaches Targeting Downstream Mechanisms of Heart Failure

Nonspecific molecular approaches to DCM target cellular abnormalities occurring in the context of HF, regardless of its cause. For example, several studies have shown that the expression of sarcoplasmic reticulum Ca^{2+}-ATPase protein (SERCA2a), a major cardiac calcium cycling protein, is consistently decreased in various forms of HF. Following an encouraging preliminary phase 2 experience, the CUPID-2 (Calcium Upregulation by Percutaneous Administration of Gene Therapy in Cardiac Disease Phase 2b) assessed the effect of SERCA2a gene transfer through infusion of AAV1/SERCA2a in 250 patients with HF and LVEF less than 35% due to an ischemic or nonischemic causes.[54] Unfortunately, there was no benefit in the treatment arm compared with placebo at 17-month follow-up. Failure has been principally attributed to limitations in the gene delivery technique. Although lack of stringent patient selection based on cause may have also played a role, a prespecified analysis did not show any interaction with the cause of HF (ischemic vs nonischemic cause). Of note, the recent randomized trial by Hammond and colleagues,[55] showing a significant improvement in LVEF following intracoronary delivery of adenovirus 5 encoding adenylyl cyclase 6 in 56 patients with HF, also included both ischemic and nonischemic causes. Adenylyl cyclase type 6, a second messenger acting as an important determinant of cardiac function, is reduced in failing hearts, and preclinical studies have shown benefits related to its increase in cardiac myocytes.[55]

With regard to attempts aimed at preventing phenotype development in DCM mutation carriers, the PRECARDIA study (PREclinical Mutation CARriers From Families With DIlated Cardiomyopathy and ACE Inhibitors, NCT01583114; see **Table 1**) involved several European centers but was terminated early because of difficult recruitment in 2016. PRECARDIA aimed to prevent DCM development with perindopril in genotype-positive phenotype-negative individuals with at least one DCM-affected family member. The study failed to show clinical benefit in the treated arm. There are several potential explanations for this failure, including the heterogeneous and unpredictable clinical expression of pathogenic and likely pathogenic mutations (even in family members with identical mutations) confronted with the limited sample size.

CHANGING SCENARIOS IN METABOLIC CARDIOMYOPATHIES: ANDERSON FABRY DISEASE

Like DMD, Anderson Fabry disease (FD) is an X-linked multisystemic lysosomal storage disorder caused by a deficiency of the enzyme α-galactosidase A, which is encoded by the GLA gene. The disease mostly affects men, but FD heterozygous women frequently show signs and symptoms of disease and may be severely affected.[56] FD leads to the progressive systematic accumulation of globotriaosylceramide (Gb3) particularly in lysosomes of the kidneys, heart, skin, and brain.[56] Two major FD phenotypes, the classic type 1 and the later-onset type 2, have been described.[56] Clinical features in classically affected male patients, with severe GLA gene mutations and a α-Gal A activity of less than 1%, include acroparesthesia, angiokeratomas, corneal dystrophy, and hypohidrosis in early childhood or adolescence, and progression to renal insufficiency, HCM, and cerebrovascular disease in adulthood.[56,57] GLA variants leading to higher residual enzyme activity can lead to an attenuated phenotype with late onset FD and relatively isolated manifestations, such as HCM, renal failure, or cryptogenic stroke at later stages in life.[58] Effective enzyme replacement therapy (ERT) has been available for FD since 2001. In addition, many alternative in vitro and in vivo therapeutic approaches, such as substrate reduction therapy, gene therapy, and exon skipping, have been experimented.[57,58] Recently, an oral chaperone treatment using the small aminosugar 1-deoxygalactonojirimycin (migalastat), obtained significant results in patients with amenable GLA gene mutations (FACETS AT1001-011; ClinicalTrials.gov Identifier: NCT00925301).[59,60] Among the 900-plus GLA gene variants reported so far (Human Gene Mutation Database professional, http://www.hgmd.org), approximately 60% are missense and many of them are potentially responsive to migalastat.[61] A chaperone is "a small molecule that enters cells and serves as a molecular framework which causes otherwise-misfolded mutant or wild type proteins to fold and route correctly within the cell."[59] Many missense variants, located out of the active site, lead to the loss of function in mutated proteins as a consequence of their degradation, or inappropriate trafficking. Such changes affect the 3-dimensional conformation of the protein. These misfolded proteins cannot pass the quality control system of the endoplasmic reticulum (ER), where they can be retained, degraded or abnormally glycosylated, and mistrafficked.[62] The concept of molecular chaperone was first introduced in 2000 by Asano and colleagues[63] and pioneered in late-onset FD patients by Frustaci and colleagues[64] with the intravenous administration of galactose. Migalastat is a pharmacologic chaperone that selectively binds the active site of the newly synthesized enzyme α-Gal A. This binding leads to the native conformation of the protein and increases the enzyme's physical stability, restoring the trafficking of the α-Gal A protein to the lysosomes, where the active enzyme can catabolize substrates[65] (**Fig. 5**). In vitro cell line experiments have widely demonstrated that α-Gal A mutant proteins carrying some of the known missense mutations can recover full-enzyme activity following migalastat administered. Orally available Migalastat has recently been licensed for FD patients carrying amenable GLA mutations.[66] Of note, in vitro studies show that chaperones can enhance the physical stability, and possibly the efficacy, of the wild-type recombinant enzymes that are commonly used for ERT.[67] A synergistic effect was confirmed in a preliminary clinical experience, suggesting that a strategy based on the coadministration of ERT and migalastat may benefit FD patients with no residual enzyme activity (NCT01218659).

NOVEL MOLECULAR TARGETS

Biotechnological and pharmacologic advances that have emerged in recent years offer new opportunities for the treatment of cardiomyopathies. The most important advances include the use on noncoding micro-RNAs (miRNAs), cell therapy, restoration of proteasome and autophagy, sodium-glucose co-transoparter-2 inhibition, and targeted DNA editing.

Noncoding Micro-RNAs

miRNAs are small noncoding RNAs involved in the regulation of cardiomyocyte function, and

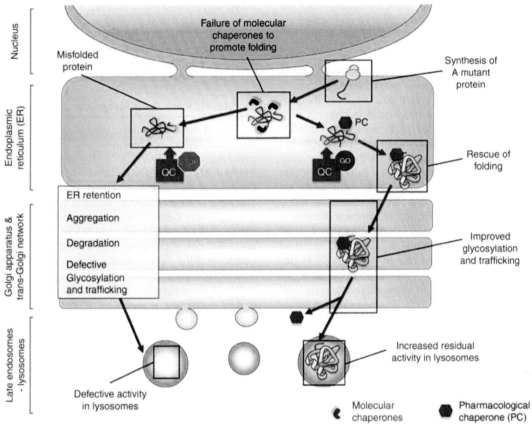

Fig. 5. Proposed mechanism of enzyme stabilization by pharmacologic chaperones. QC, quality control. (*From* Parenti G, Andria G, Valenzano KJ. Pharmacological chaperone therapy: preclinical development, clinical translation, and prospects for the treatment of lysosomal storage disorders. Mol Ther 2015;23(7):1140; with permission.)

changes in their expression are implicated in the pathophysiology of several heart diseases, including HCM and DCM.[68] The expression of several miRNAs is altered in the myocardium of HCM patients, depending on the stage and the severity of disease expression.[69] Moreover, the plasma level of specific miRNAs (eg, miR29a) is increased in patients with symptomatic HCM and severe fibrosis, representing possible biomarkers of adverse outcome.[70] Furthermore, altered levels of circulating miRNAs have been associated with severe arrhythmias in patients with arrhythmogenic cardiomyopathy.[71] MiRNAs-based therapies for cardiomyopathies aim to modulate the expression of these noncoding RNAs in the cardiomyocyte, by antagonizing the function of pro-hypertrophic and profibrotic miRNAs (by synthetic miRNAs or "antimiRs") or by mimicking the effects of endogenous miRNAs that antagonize hypertrophy and cardiac remodeling.[72] A recent study in animal models showed that inhibition of miR-208b improved cardiac function in titin-

based DCM.[73] miRNAs can be naturally transported in biological fluids and delivered to cells, making them good targets for therapy; however, optimization of delivery strategies must be achieved to obtain a cardiac-specific effect (eg, by using nanoparticles).[74] In addition, long non-coding RNAs are also emerging as possible regulators of cardiac function and are being implicated in HCM and DCM.[75] Strategies based on long noncoding RNA to modulate angiogenesis in cardiac diseases have being evaluated in vitro[76]; however, their use as therapeutic targets is limited by their large molecular weight, requiring specialized delivery strategies. Finally, small interfering RNAs (siRNAs) are oligonucleotides that can reduce the expression of target proteins by selectively inhibiting the transcription of specific mRNAs. In a mouse model of HCM, silencing of the mutated allele through viral-mediated cardiac delivery of a specific siRNA completely prevented the development of the LVH.[18] The development of siRNA-based drugs is particularly advanced: pioneering clinical studies include agents that reduce liver transthyretin (TTR) synthesis for the treatment of cardiac TTR amyloidosis.[77]

Cell Therapy

Therapeutic strategies involving the use of cells to repair the damaged heart or to improve its contractile function have been used in patients with ischemic heart disease with conflicting results.[78] Notably, bone marrow–derived mesenchymal stem cells (MSCs) delivered to the myocardium via transendocardial catheter-based injection improved symptoms in patients with ischemic HF.[79] More recently, the POSEIDON-DCM study demonstrated the efficacy of allogenic MSCs in patients with inherited DCM: treatment with MSCs increased ejection fraction and reduced HF symptoms and the rate of events in DCM patients.[80] However, the large-scale applicability of such an approach in clinical practice is still unresolved.

Proteasome and Autophagy

The ubiquitin-proteasome system (UPS) plays an essential role in protein quality control and programmed cell death.[81] Proteasome impairment is a determinant of hypertrophy, myocardial ischemia, and HF,[82] and LV dysfunction is a frequent complication of proteasome inhibitors (such as bortezomib) in patients with cancer.[83] UPS impairment accelerates disease progression by several mechanisms: (a) accumulation of proteins involved in hypertrophic signaling (eg, calcineurin) or apoptosis (eg, p53); (b) accumulation of unfolded/misfolded proteins in the ER, leading to reduced protein synthesis and apoptosis; (c) persistence of dysfunctional ion channel proteins, contributing to electrical instability and arrhythmias.[84,85] Pharmacologic stimulation of the proteasome would be beneficial for the treatment of cardiomyopathies.[86] For example, proteasome function is selectively impaired in HCM caused by cMyBP-C mutations: the mutated/truncated protein is degraded by the proteasome at a faster rate than the wild-type protein, leading to UPS overload and dysfunction.[84] To date, however, no selective proteasome activator is available. An indirect way to enhance proteasome function is to target protein kinase Gm, for example, by the PDE5 inhibitor sildenafil.[87] Indeed, sildenafil is known to improve LV diastolic and systolic function in failing patients and animal models,[88] but remains to be tested in HCM and DCM. Finally, an indirect consequence of proteasome dysfunction in cardiomyopathies is the overload of the other cellular protein degradation system, the autophagy-lysosomal pathway, leading to intracellular accumulation of residual bodies, as shown in the hearts of HCM mice.[89] Interestingly, restoration of autophagy flux with rapamycin or caloric restriction partially rescued cardiomyopathy in transgenic mice with cMyBP-C mutations.[89]

Sodium-Glucose Co-transoparter 2 Inhibition

The novel oral antidiabetic agents, empagliflozin and canagliflozin, are inhibitors of sodium glucose cotransporter 2 (SGLT2).[90] Of note, both the EMPA-REG OUTCOME trial ([Empagliflozin] Cardiovascular Outcome Event Trial in Type 2 Diabetes Mellitus Patients) and the CANVAS trial (Canagliflozin Cardiovascular Assessment Study) demonstrated significant reductions in mortality and HF hospitalization in patients with type 2 diabetes mellitus and cardiovascular disease.[90] Therefore, even though the cardioprotective action of these agents is incompletely understood, SGLT2 inhibition is seen as a very promising strategy for HF of any cause. SGLT2 inhibition induces natriuresis and osmotic diuresis, causing plasma volume contraction and reduced preload; moreover, it decreases blood pressure, arterial stiffness, and cardiac afterload, leading to improvement of myocardial blood flow.[90] Large clinical trials with SGLT2 inhibitors are currently investigating the possible use of SGLT2 inhibitors in patients with HF in the absence of diabetes. No specific trials have been programmed specifically for patients with inherited DCM, but DCM patients will be included in the ongoing studies. Recently, SGLT2 inhibition was shown to directly target cardiomyocytes by blocking the H^+/Na^+ exchanger (NHE) on the cell membrane.[91] Inhibition of the NHE may result in lower cardiomyocyte Na^+ concentration, in turn ameliorating intracellular Ca^{2+} handling. As intracellular Na^+ is abnormally increased in HCM cardiomyocytes, Na^+ reduction by SGLT2 inhibitors may provide specific clinical benefit in this condition.[92]

Targeted DNA-Editing

Genome-editing tools, including zinc finger nucleases, transcription activator-like effector nucleases, and clustered regularly interspaced short palindromic repeats (CRISPR)/CRISPR-associated 9 (Cas9) systems, are emerging as valid biotechnology approaches to obtain germline and somatic genomic manipulation in cells and organisms for multiple purposes (eg, creation of knockout models, introduction of mutations, insertion of transgenes).[93] Genome editing is being extensively used in cardiovascular research, ranging from lipid metabolism to electrophysiology and cardiomyopathies, contributing to the creation of novel cellular and animal models.[93] Moreover, genome-editing approaches have opened the door to a new class of therapies acting at the DNA level (see **Table 2**). As previously mentioned, CRISPR-Cas9 technology was successfully used to correct a cMyBP-C mutation in in vitro fertilized embryos.[20] The first attempt to use genome-editing technology to achieve a cardio-specific correction of a cardiomyopathy-related mutation was achieved in mice carrying a DMD mutation.[94] SaCas9 (CRISPR-associated protein 9 from *Staphylococcus aureus*) was packaged into a cardio-selective AAV with RNA constructs and delivered in vivo in neonatal mice to obtain an effective excision of exon 23 of DMD gene in dystrophic mice: this led to a complete prevention of the cardiac phenotype in the absence of extracardiac effects. Attempts to use this technology to treat other cardiomyopathies are ongoing.

SUMMARY

Precision medicine is becoming a reality in many areas of cardiovascular medicine, including cardiomyopathies. Although the clinical impact of tailored interventions is still limited, the breadth and scope of ongoing research in the field is unprecedented and proceeding at impressive speed. The unique and complex profile of myocardial diseases, as well as their unfavorable epidemiology, represents major challenges requiring a spectrum of solutions ranging from innovative molecules to novel trial designs, whose benefit will plausibly expand to other fields of cardiology. If this can be achieved, the coming years appear full of promise for cardiomyopathy patients and their families.

ACKNOWLEDGMENTS

This work was supported by the Italian Ministry of Health (Left ventricular hypertrophy in aortic valve disease and hypertrophic cardiomyopathy: genetic basis, biophysical correlates and viral therapy models) RF-2013-02356787, and NET-2011-02347173 (Mechanisms and treatment of coronary microvascular dysfunction in patients with genetic or secondary left ventricular hypertrophy); by Telethon Italy (GGP13162); and by the ToRSADE project (FAS-Salute 2014, Regione Toscana).

REFERENCES

1. Rapezzi C, Arbustini E, Caforio AL, et al. Diagnostic work-up in cardiomyopathies: bridging the gap between clinical phenotypes and final diagnosis. A position statement from the ESC Working Group on Myocardial and Pericardial Diseases. Eur Heart J 2013;34:1448–58.

2. Maron BJ, Rowin EJ, Casey SA, et al. How hypertrophic cardiomyopathy became a contemporary treatable genetic disease with low mortality: shaped by 50 years of clinical research and practice. JAMA Cardiol 2016;1:98–105.

3. Ammirati E, Contri R, Coppini R, et al. Pharmacological treatment of hypertrophic cardiomyopathy: current practice and novel perspectives. Eur J Heart Fail 2016;18(9):1106–18.

4. Van Der Velden J, Ho CY, Tardiff JC, et al. Research priorities in sarcomeric cardiomyopathies. Cardiovasc Res 2015;105(4):449–56.

5. Olivotto I, Hellawell JL, Farzaneh-Far R, et al. Novel approach targeting the complex pathophysiology of hypertrophic cardiomyopathy. Circ Heart Fail 2016; 9(3):e002764.

6. Semsarian C, Ingles J, Maron MS, et al. New perspectives on the prevalence of hypertrophic cardiomyopathy. J Am Coll Cardiol 2015;65(12):1249–54.

7. Bhatt DL, Mehta C. Adaptive designs for clinical trials. N Engl J Med 2016;375(1):65–74.

8. Elliott PM, Anastasakis A, Borger MA, et al. 2014 ESC guidelines on diagnosis and management of hypertrophic cardiomyopathy: the Task Force for the Diagnosis and Management of Hypertrophic Cardiomyopathy of the European Society of Cardiology (ESC). Eur Heart J 2014;35:2733–79.

9. Ho CY, Lakdawala NK, Cirino AL, et al. Diltiazem treatment for pre-clinical hypertrophic cardiomyopathy sarcomere mutation carriers: a pilot randomized trial to modify disease expression. JACC Heart Fail 2015;3:180–8.

10. Sommese RF, Sung J, Nag S, et al. Molecular consequences of the R453C hypertrophic cardiomyopathy mutation on human β-cardiac myosin motor function. Proc Natl Acad Sci U S A 2013;110(31):12607–12.

11. Green EM, Wakimoto H, Anderson RL, et al. A small-molecule inhibitor of sarcomere contractility suppresses hypertrophic cardiomyopathy in mice. Science 2016;351(6273):617–21.

12. Horowitz JD, Chirkov YY. Perhexiline and hypertrophic cardiomyopathy: a new horizon for metabolic modulation. Circulation 2010;122:1547–9.

13. Abozguia K, Elliott P, McKenna W, et al. Metabolic modulator perhexiline corrects energy deficiency and improves exercise capacity in symptomatic hypertrophic cardiomyopathy. Circulation 2010;122: 1562–9.

14. Spoladore R, Maron MS, D'Amato R, et al. Pharmacological treatment options for hypertrophic cardiomyopathy: high time for evidence. Eur Heart J 2012;33:1724–33.

15. Olivotto I, Camici PG, Merlini PA, et al. Efficacy of Ranolazine in Patients With Symptomatic Hypertrophic Cardiomyopathy: The RESTYLE-HCM Randomized,

Double-Blind, Placebo-Controlled Study. Circulation: Heart Failure 2018;11(1):e004124.

16. Ferrantini C, Coppini R, Pioner JM, et al. Pathogenesis of hypertrophic cardiomyopathy is mutation rather than disease specific: a comparison of the cardiac troponin T E163R and R92Q mouse models. J Am Heart Assoc 2017;6(7) [pii: e005407].

17. Rajamani S, El-Bizri N, Liu G, et al. Abstract 16790: anti-arrhythmic properties of a novel cardiac late Na+ current inhibitor, GS-6615, in a mouse model of long QT type 3. Circulation 2014;130:A16790.

18. Jiang J, Wakimoto H, Seidman JG, et al. Allele-specific silencing of mutant Myh6 transcripts in mice suppresses hypertrophic cardiomyopathy. Science 2013;342(6154):111–4.

19. Mearini G, Stimpel D, Geertz B, et al. Mybpc3 gene therapy for neonatal cardiomyopathy enables long-term disease prevention in mice. Nat Commun 2014;5:5515.

20. Ma H, Marti-Gutierrez N, Park SW, et al. Correction of a pathogenic gene mutation in human embryos. Nature 2017;548(7668):413–9.

21. Lim DS, Lutucuta S, Bachireddy P, et al. Angiotensin II blockade reverses myocardial fibrosis in a transgenic mouse model of human hypertrophic cardiomyopathy. Circulation 2001;103:789–91.

22. Ho CY, McMurray JJ, Cirino AL, et al. Valsartan for attenuating disease evolution in early sarcomeric hypertrophic cardiomyopathy: the design of the valsartan for attenuating disease evolution in early sarcomeric hypertrophic cardiomyopathy (VANISH) trial. Am Heart J 2017;187:145–55.

23. Shimada YJ, Passeri JJ, Baggish AL, et al. Effects of losartan on left ventricular hypertrophy and fibrosis in patients with nonobstructive hypertrophic cardiomyopathy. JACC Heart Fail 2013;1(6):480–7.

24. Axelsson A, Iversen K, Vejlstrup N, et al. Efficacy and safety of the angiotensin II receptor blocker losartan for hypertrophic cardiomyopathy: the INHERIT randomised, double-blind, placebo-controlled trial. Lancet Diabetes Endocrinol 2015; 3(2):123–31.

25. Lombardi R, Rodriguez G, Chen SN, et al. Resolution of established cardiac hypertrophy and fibrosis and prevention of systolic dysfunction in a transgenic rabbit model of human cardiomyopathy through thiol-sensitive mechanisms. Circulation 2009;119:1398–407.

26. Senthil V, Chen SN, Tsybouleva N, et al. Prevention of cardiac hypertrophy by atorvastatin in a transgenic rabbit model of human hypertrophic cardiomyopathy. Circ Res 2005;97:285–92.

27. Nagueh SF, Lombardi R, Tan Y, et al. Atorvastatin and cardiac hypertrophy and function in hypertrophic cardiomyopathy: a pilot study. Eur J Clin Invest 2010;40:976–83.

28. Japp AG, Gulati A, Cook SA, et al. The diagnosis and evaluation of dilated cardiomyopathy. J Am Coll Cardiol 2016;67:2996–3010.

29. Køber L, Thune JJ, Nielsen JC, et al. Defibrillator implantation in patients with nonischemic systolic heart failure. N Engl J Med 2016;375(13):1221–30.

30. Castelli G, Fornaro A, Ciaccheri M, et al. Improving survival rates of patients with idiopathic dilated cardiomyopathy in tuscany over three decades: impact of evidence-based management. Circ Heart Fail 2013;6(5):913–21.

31. Burke MA, Cook SA, Seidman JG, et al. Clinical and mechanistic insights into the genetics of cardiomyopathy. J Am Coll Cardiol 2016;68:2871–86.

32. Herman DS, Lam L, Taylor MR, et al. Truncations of titin causing dilated cardiomyopathy. N Engl J Med 2012;366:619–28.

33. Tayal U, Newsome S, Buchan R, et al. Phenotype and clinical outcomes of titin cardiomyopathy. J Am Coll Cardiol 2017;70:2264–74.

34. Guo W, Schafer S, Greaser ML, et al. RBM20, a gene for hereditary cardiomyopathy, regulates titin splicing. Nat Med 2012;18:766–73.

35. Schmitt JP, Kamisago M, Asahi M, et al. Dilated cardiomyopathy and heart failure caused by a mutation in phospholamban. Science 2003;299:1410–3.

36. Fatkin D, MacRae C, Sasaki T, et al. Missense mutations in the rod domain of the lamin A/C gene as causes of dilated cardiomyopathy and conduction-system disease. N Engl J Med 1999;341:1715–24.

37. Meune C, Van Berlo JH, Anselme F, et al. Primary prevention of sudden death in patients with lamin A/C gene mutations. N Engl J Med 2006;354: 209–10.

38. Captur G, Arbustini E, Bonne G, et al. Lamin and the heart. Heart 2017. https://doi.org/10.1136/heartjnl-2017-312338.

39. Mann SA, Castro ML, Ohanian M, et al. R222Q SCN5A mutation is associated with reversible ventricular ectopy and dilated cardiomyopathy. J Am Coll Cardiol 2012;60:1566–73.

40. Hoffman EP, Brown RH, Kunkel LM. Dystrophin: the protein product of the Duchenne muscular dystrophy locus. Cell 1987;51(6):919–28.

41. Nakamura A. Moving towards successful exon-skipping therapy for Duchenne muscular dystrophy. J Hum Genet 2017;62(10):871–6.

42. Chamberlain JR, Chamberlain JS. Progress toward gene therapy for Duchenne muscular dystrophy. Mol Ther 2017;25(5):1125–31.

43. Koenig M, Monaco AP, Kunkel LM. The complete sequence of dystrophin predicts a rod-shaped cytoskeletal protein. Cell 1988;53(2):219–28.

44. Nance ME, Hakim CH, Yang NN, et al. Nanotherapy for Duchenne muscular dystrophy. Wiley Interdiscip Rev Nanomed Nanobiotechnol 2017. [Epub ahead of print].

45. Bello L, Pegoraro E. Genetic diagnosis as a tool for personalized treatment of Duchenne muscular dystrophy. Acta Myol 2016;35(3):122.

46. Bajek A, Porowinska D, Kloskowski T, et al. Cell therapy in Duchenne muscular dystrophy treatment: clinical trials overview. Crit Rev Eukaryot Gene Expr 2015;25(1):1–11.

47. Nelson CE, Hakim CH, Ousterout DG, et al. In vivo genome editing improves muscle function in a mouse model of Duchenne muscular dystrophy. Science 2016;351(6271):403–7.

48. Aartsma-Rus A, Fokkema I, Verschuuren J, et al. Theoretic applicability of antisense-mediated exon skipping for Duchenne muscular dystrophy mutations. Hum Mutat 2009;30(3):293–9.

49. Cirak S, Arechavala-Gomeza V, Guglieri M, et al. Exon skipping and dystrophin restoration in patients with Duchenne muscular dystrophy after systemic phosphorodiamidate morpholino oligomer treatment: an open-label, phase 2, dose-escalation study. Lancet 2011;378(9791):595–605.

50. Van Deutekom JC, Janson AA, Ginjaar IB, et al. Local dystrophin restoration with antisense oligonucleotide PRO051. N Engl J Med 2007;357(26): 2677–86.

51. McDonald CM, Campbell C, Torricelli RE, et al. Ataluren in patients with nonsense mutation Duchenne muscular dystrophy (ACT DMD): a multicentre, randomised, double-blind, placebo-controlled, phase 3 trial. Lancet 2017;390(10101):1489–98.

52. Kamdar F, Garry DJ. Dystrophin-deficient cardiomyopathy. J Am Coll Cardiol 2016;67:2533–46.

53. Syed YY. Eteplirsen: first global approval. Drugs 2016;76(17):1699–704.

54. Greenberg B, Butler J, Felker GM. Calcium upregulation by percutaneous administration of gene therapy in patients with cardiac disease (CUPID 2): a randomised, multinational, double-blind, placebo-controlled, phase 2b trial. Lancet 2016;387: 1178–86.

55. Hammond H, Penny WF, Traverse JH. Intracoronary gene transfer of adenylyl cyclase 6 in patients with heart failure. JAMA Cardiol 2016;1:163–71.

56. Germain DP. Fabry disease. Orphanet J Rare Dis 2010;5:30.

57. Guérard N, Oder D, Nordbeck P, et al. Lucerastat, an iminosugar for substrate reduction therapy: tolerability, pharmacodynamics, and pharmacokinetics in patients with Fabry disease on enzyme replacement. Clin Pharmacol Ther 2017. https://doi.org/10.1002/cpt.790.

58. Huang J, Khan A, Au BC, et al. Lentivector iterations and pre-clinical scale-up/toxicity testing: targeting mobilized CD34+ cells for correction of Fabry disease. Mol Ther Methods Clin Dev 2017;5:241–58.

59. Germain DP, Hughes DA, Nicholls K, et al. Treatment of Fabry's disease with the pharmacologic chaperone migalastat. N Engl J Med 2016;375(6): 545–55.

60. Hughes DA, Nicholls K, Shankar SP, et al. Oral pharmacological chaperone migalastat compared with enzyme replacement therapy in Fabry disease: 18-month results from the randomised phase III ATTRACT study. J Med Genet 2017;54:288–96.

61. Filoni C, Caciotti A, Carraresi L, et al. Functional studies of new GLA gene mutations leading to conformational Fabry disease. Biochim Biophys Acta 2010;1802(2):247–52.

62. Parenti G, Fecarotta S, La Marca G, et al. A chaperone enhances blood α-glucosidase activity in Pompe disease patients treated with enzyme replacement therapy. Mol Ther 2014;22(11): 2004–12.

63. Asano N, Ishii S, Kizu H, et al. In vitro inhibition and intracellular enhancement of lysosomal alpha-galactosidase A activity in Fabry lymphoblasts by 1-deoxygalactonojirimycin and its derivatives. FEBS J 2000;267(13):4179–86.

64. Frustaci A, Chimenti C, Ricci R, et al. Improvement in cardiac function in the cardiac variant of Fabry's disease with galactose-infusion therapy. N Engl J Med 2001;345(1):25–32.

65. Parenti G, Andria G, Valenzano KJ. Pharmacological chaperone therapy: preclinical development, clinical translation, and prospects for the treatment of lysosomal storage disorders. Mol Ther 2015;23(7): 1138–48.

66. Benjamin ER, Della Valle MC, Wu X, et al. The validation of pharmacogenetics for the identification of Fabry patients to be treated with migalastat. Genet Med 2017;19(4):430–8.

67. Porto C, Pisani A, Rosa M, et al. Synergy between the pharmacological chaperone 1-deoxygalactonojirimycin and the human recombinant alpha galactosidase A in cultured fibroblasts from patients with Fabry disease. J Inherit Metab Dis 2012;35(3): 513–20.

68. Roma-Rodrigues C, Raposo LR, Fernandes AR. MicroRNAs based therapy of hypertrophic cardiomyopathy: the road traveled so far. Biomed Res Int 2015;2015:983290.

69. Kuster DW, Mulders J, Folkert J, et al. MicroRNA transcriptome profiling in cardiac tissue of hypertrophic cardiomyopathy patients with MYBPC3 mutations. J Mol Cell Cardiol 2013;65:59–66.

70. Roncarati R, Anselmi CV, Losi MA, et al. Circulating miR-29a, among other up-regulated microRNAs, is the only biomarker for both hypertrophy and fibrosis in patients with hypertrophic cardiomyopathy. J Am Coll Cardiol 2014;63(9):920–7.

71. Yamada S, Hsiao YW, Chang SL, et al. Circulating microRNAs in arrhythmogenic right ventricular cardiomyopathy with ventricular arrhythmia. Europace 2017. https://doi.org/10.1093/europace/eux289.

72. Van Rooij E, Kauppinen S. Development of microRNA therapeutics is coming of age. EMBO Mol Med 2014;6(7):851–64.

73. Zhou Q, Schötterl S, Backes D, et al. Inhibition of miR-208b improves cardiac function in titin-based dilated cardiomyopathy. Int J Cardiol 2017;230: 634–41.

74. Baptista PV. Gold nanobeacons: a potential nanotheranostics platform. Nanomedicine (Lond) 2014; 9(15):2247–50.

75. Kitow J, Derda AA, Beermann J, et al. Mitochondrial long noncoding RNAs as blood based biomarkers for cardiac remodeling in patients with hypertrophic cardiomyopathy. Am J Physiol Heart Circ Physiol 2016;311(3):H707–12.

76. Leisegang MS, Fork C, Josipovic I, et al. Long noncoding RNA MANTIS facilitates endothelial angiogenic function. Circulation 2017;136(1):65–79.

77. Poller W, Dimmeler S, Heymans S, et al. Non-coding RNAs in cardiovascular diseases: diagnostic and therapeutic perspectives. Eur Heart J 2017. https://doi.org/10.1093/eurheartj/ehx165.

78. Madonna R, Van Laake LW, Davidson SM, et al. Position paper of the European Society of Cardiology Working Group Cellular Biology of the Heart: cell-based therapies for myocardial repair and regeneration in ischemic heart disease and heart failure. Eur Heart J 2016;37(23):1789–98.

79. Hare JM, Fishman JE, Gerstenblith G, et al. Comparison of allogeneic vs autologous bone marrow–derived mesenchymal stem cells delivered by trans-endocardial injection in patients with ischemic cardiomyopathy: the POSEIDON randomized trial. JAMA 2012;308(22):2369–79.

80. Hare JM, DiFede DL, Rieger AC, et al. Randomized comparison of allogeneic versus autologous mesenchymal stem cells for nonischemic dilated cardiomyopathy: POSEIDON-DCM trial. J Am Coll Cardiol 2017;69(5):526–37.

81. Gilda JE, Gomes AV. Proteasome dysfunction in cardiomyopathies. J Physiol 2017;595(12): 4051–71.

82. Voortman J, Giaccone G. Severe reversible cardiac failure after bortezomib treatment combined with chemotherapy in a non-small cell lung cancer patient: a case report. BMC Cancer 2006;6(1):129.

83. Schlossarek S, Frey N, Carrier L. Ubiquitin-proteasome system and hereditary cardiomyopathies. J Mol Cell Cardiol 2014;71:25–31.

84. Bahrudin U, Morikawa K, Takeuchi A, et al. Impairment of ubiquitin–proteasome system by E334K cMyBPC modifies channel proteins, leading to electrophysiological dysfunction. J Mol Biol 2011;413(4): 857–78.

85. Li J, Horak KM, Su H, et al. Enhancement of proteasomal function protects against cardiac proteinopathy and ischemia/reperfusion injury in mice. J Clin Invest 2011;121(9):3689.

86. Ranek MJ, Terpstra EJ, Li J, et al. Protein kinase g positively regulates proteasome-mediated degradation of misfolded proteins. Circulation 2013;128(4): 365–76.

87. Takimoto E, Champion HC, Li M, et al. Chronic inhibition of cyclic GMP phosphodiesterase 5A prevents and reverses cardiac hypertrophy. Nat Med 2005; 11(2):214–22.

88. Schlossarek S, Mearini G, Carrier L. Cardiac myosin-binding protein C in hypertrophic cardiomyopathy: mechanisms and therapeutic opportunities. J Mol Cell Cardiol 2011;50(4):613–20.

89. Singh SR, Zech AT, Geertz B, et al. Activation of autophagy ameliorates cardiomyopathy in Mybpc3-targeted knockin mice. Circ Heart Fail 2017;10(10):e004140.

90. Lytvyn Y, Bjornstad P, Udell JA, et al. Sodium glucose cotransporter-2 inhibition in heart failure: potential mechanisms, clinical applications, and summary of clinical trials. Circulation 2017;136(17): 1643–58.

91. Baartscheer A, Schumacher CA, Wüst RC, et al. Empagliflozin decreases myocardial cytoplasmic Na+ through inhibition of the cardiac Na+/H+ exchanger in rats and rabbits. Diabetologia 2017;60(3):568–73.

92. Coppini R, Ferrantini C, Yao L, et al. Late sodium current inhibition reverses electro-mechanical dysfunction in human hypertrophic cardiomyopathy. Circulation 2013;127(5):575–84.

93. Strong A, Musunuru K. Genome editing in cardiovascular diseases. Nat Rev Cardiol 2017;14(1): 11–20.

94. Refaey ME, Xu L, Gao Y, et al. In vivo genome editing restores dystrophin expression and cardiac function in dystrophic mice. Circ Res 2017;121(8): 923–9.

Gene Editing and Gene-Based Therapeutics for Cardiomyopathies

Joyce C. Ohiri, BS, Elizabeth M. McNally, MD, PhD*

KEYWORDS

- Genetic mutations • Genetic correction • Gene editing • Antisense oligonucleotides
- Cardiomyopathy • Heart failure • Muscular dystrophy

KEY POINTS

- Genetic editing targeting DNA sequences can correct underlying genetic mutations.
- Viral vectors are used to deliver gene editing machinery to the heart.
- Antisense oligonucleotides target RNA to modulate splicing, and this approach requires repeated dosing.

INTRODUCTION

Cardiomyopathy and heart failure are under genetic influence. Genetic correction technologies are rapidly emerging, providing the tools to correct underlying genetic defects responsible for human disease, including cardiomyopathy. Gene-editing strategies like clustered regularly interspaced short palindromic repeats (CRISPR/Cas9) act on DNA. There are also RNA-targeted approaches, including antisense oligonucleotides or even gene editing, which are used to suppress mutations or promote expression of functional molecules. Genetic correction strategies are designed to reverse specific mutations responsible for disease, or these same methods can also be applied to modulate normal sequences in order to improve heart function. Most genetic correction approaches are gene and mutation specific, and therefore require knowledge of the underlying genetic mutations responsible for cardiomyopathy and heart failure, further underscoring the importance of genetic diagnosis.

TECHNICAL ADVANCES ENABLING GENETIC EDITING IN DNA

Tools for genetic engineering remain at the crux of scientific discovery and are poised for therapeutic application in heart failure. The Human Genome Project, and the subsequent efforts to define human genetic variation using larger scale efforts, have revolutionized the way in which heart failure and cardiomyopathy are approached.[1–3] Simultaneous with these efforts, the Xenopus-derived zinc finger nuclease (ZFN) emerged as an early technology to change genome sequences.[4] This DNA-binding motif was designed to recognize DNA sequences with high specificity,[5] but required engineering protein motifs to recognize DNA sequences of interest. Despite the broad application of these engineered nucleases for gene correction, expansion of ZNF use was limited by an inability to target complex sequences as well as issues related to sequence specificity. Yet, ZNF served as a gateway for the development of new and improved gene-editing technologies.

Center for Genetic Medicine, Northwestern University Feinberg School of Medicine, Chicago, IL 60611, USA
* Corresponding author. Northwestern Center for Genetic Medicine, 303 East Superior Street, Lurie 7-123, Chicago, IL 60611.
E-mail address: Elizabeth.mcnally@northwestern.edu

Heart Failure Clin 14 (2018) 179–188
https://doi.org/10.1016/j.hfc.2017.12.006
1551-7136/18/© 2017 Elsevier Inc. All rights reserved.

Transcription activator-like effector nucleases (TALENS) represented an advance for genomic engineering.[6,7] These nucleases are engineered constructs that contain a DNA-binding domain and a nonspecific nuclease domain.[8] TALENS generate double strand breaks (DSBs) at specific sites of interest within a given DNA sequence, which are subsequently repaired by nonhomologous end joining (NHEJ). This process induces the formation of insertion and deletion mutations. Unlike ZFNs, TALENs' comparatively fast and easy construction allowed for a more precise and efficient method for genomic targeting.[9] The emergence of TALENs advanced pre-existing methods for gene editing, and these nucleases served as a guide for the onset of innovative tools for gene-based therapies.

Found in both bacteria and archaea, CRISPR/Cas9 emerged as the next generation in genome editing as a system that modifies DNA by generating site-specific cleavage events, which may then be followed by a template-driven repair process.[4,10] With a template-driven repair process, specific sequences can be changed, or new sequences can be inserted or deleted. Similar to previous mechanisms, CRISPR/Cas9 functions by creating DSBs at precise sites within the DNA. The site specificity is driven by guide RNAs, which use this homology to carry the Cas9 nuclease to specific sites. After cleavage by Cas9, DSBs can be repaired by NHEJ, which most commonly results in deletions of varying size and length. Alternatively, in the presence of a template, homology-directed repair (HDR) occurs, in which the DSB is repaired to resemble the template. HDR can be exploited to yield site-specific precise genetic correction, for example, from a mutation to a normal allele. HDR can also be exploited to add sequences of interest or more precisely delete selected regions.[11] In contrast to NHEJ, an error-prone system that fuses together blunt ends of DNA without the use of a repair template, HDR is more accurate by involving the recombination of a homologous template strand. However, HDR is a less efficient method of DSB repair compared with NHEJ. CRISPR/Cas9 was first described in 2012 and then adapted for its use in mammalian cells.[12–14] Since this discovery, CRISPR/Cas9 has been making headways in genomic engineering, providing useful tools in the laboratory setting and also in its development for therapeutic genetic correction.

DNA GENE EDITING USING CLUSTERED REGULARLY INTERSPACED SHORT PALINDROMIC REPEATS/CAS9

In bacteria, the CRISPR/Cas9 system is an endonuclease important for cleaving viral DNA. The adaptation of this endonuclease system

ultimately relies on guide RNAs to direct the endonuclease, Cas9, to specific sequence sites that are then cleaved. Single-guide RNA sequences (sgRNAs) are short synthetic RNA molecules that direct the Cas9 endonuclease protein to generate DSBs near the site of interest (**Fig. 1**). The precision of this cleavage depends on the accuracy of the sgRNAs. The region of target homology in sgRNAs is approximately 20 base pairs, and even single base pair mismatch reduces target engagement. It is possible to utilize more than a single sgRNA (eg, to create more than one cleavage). However, a drawback of using more than a single sgRNA is decreased efficiency, because guides must find their cognate target, and an increased number of potential off-target effects may result.[15] An additional limitation of this technology is the long-term expression of Cas9 nuclease that can increase toxicity through multiple mechanisms including off-target mutations. Modifications to guide RNAs or using Cas9 nickases, which generate single-strand DNA breaks instead of double-strand DNA breaks, can reduce off-target mutations.[16] Furthermore, destabilizing domains can be added to Cas9 to provide an additional level of regulation, whereby the Cas9 can be inactivated to reduce off-target effects by limiting the lifespan of Cas9 activity.[17]

The small size of Cas9 contributes to the scalable nature of its application, making gene delivery by viral vectors possible. Cas9 endonucleases differ in size and functionality.[18] *Staphylococcus aureus* Cas9 (called SaCas9) is 1 kb smaller than Cas9 from *Streptococcus pyogenes* Cas9,[19] providing a more compact Cas9. Additionally, the longer CRISPR RNA spacer sequence of *Neisseria meningitidis* Cas9 (referred to as NmCas9) limits its targeting range, but decreases off-target activity.[20] *Streptococcus thermophiles* (StCas9) has proven to be a more specific form of Cas9, albeit less efficient than SpCas9.[21] In tandem with the findings of new Cas9 species, ongoing studies are exploring delivery channels as a means for better transportation of these molecules intracellularly.[22]

APPLICATION OF GENE EDITING IN CARDIOMYOPATHY

There are many contemplated applications of gene editing for treating heart failure. One use of gene editing is aimed at correcting underlying genetic mutations responsible for causing cardiomyopathy. Cardiomyopathies are often attributed to genetic mutations resulting in familial or inherited forms of cardiomyopathy. Hypertrophic cardiomyopathy (HCM) is often linked to sarcomere

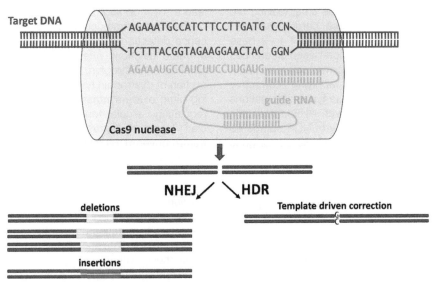

Fig. 1. CRISPR/Cas9 for gene editing. CRISPR/Cas9 is a bacterially- derived system that can be applied to specifically modify the mammalian genome. A guide RNA (*green*) is used to carry the Cas9 nuclease to a region of homology, dictated by an approximately 20 base pair region within the guide that recognizes the complementary sequences in the target DNA. Cas9 then creates a double-stranded break that is then ligated using NHEJ, generating insertions or deletions of varying sizes. Alternatively, in the presence of a template, HDR can be used to generate site-specific nucleotide changes in the target DNA.

gene mutations.[23] Dilated cardiomyopathy (DCM) is far more heterogeneous, with mutations in more than 100 genes.[24] Arrhythmogenic right ventricular cardiomyopathy (ARVC or AVC), restrictive cardiomyopathy (RCM), and left ventricular noncompaction cardiomyopathy (LVNC) each have a significant genetic component as well.[25] For each of these genetic cardiomyopathies, autosomal-dominant mutations are the most frequent mode of inheritance, although X-linked recessive, autosomal recessive, and mitochondrial inheritance also contribute. The most common genetic mutations linked to cardiomyopathies are small mutations, either single nucleotide variants (SNVs) or small insertions/deletions (indels), on the order of 1 to 30 base pairs. SNVs can result in the substitution of 1 amino acid for another, referred to as nonsynonymous SNVs (nsSNV), or result in the loss of a stop codon or insertion of a new premature stop codon (stop loss or stop gain SNVs, respectively).

Indels can produce in-frame or out-of-frame effects on the protein they encode. In-frame deletions produce internally truncated, but often functional proteins. Out-of-frame deletions may or may not be associated with residual protein expression depending on the degree of nonsense-mediated decay, which reduces the amount of mRNA, and the stability of the amino-terminal protein domains. Similarly, premature stop codons or

loss of stop codons each can result in varying degrees of residual protein expression. Predicting the effect of premature stop codons and out-of-frame mutations on residual protein expression is not straightforward and highly dependent on the protein's normal structure and function. Even small amounts of amino-terminal protein expression can result in gain-of-function, dominant negative activity. As gene correction strategies move forward to treat genetic cardiomyopathies, it is critically important to determine the precise mode of action of a given mutation, as off-target effects of gene editing could render the molecular pathology worse. For example, genetic editing that shifts an in-frame mutation to an out-of-frame mutation could result in dominant negative activity, thus making the outcome worse. At present, most gene editing results in multiple events that differ from cell to cell. Although HDR may be intended to substitute a single amino acid for another, many cells may actually have undergone NHEJ, resulting in a range of results within the heart.

In addition to ensuring high fidelity of genetic correction of the mutant gene, it is important that there is specificity for the mutant gene to avoid introducing unwanted mutations into the normal gene copy. The application of gene editing to an autosomal-dominant disease like most cardiomyopathy mutations would require correcting the mutated copy and at the same time, leaving the normal copy intact. Because cardiomyopathy-causing mutations often span only 1 to 2 base pairs, this leaves little sequence-based differences between the mutant and normal copy, necessitating tight specificity in applying corrective technologies. Correcting these types of mutations is likely to require HDR over NHEJ. With the comparatively lower efficiency of HDR compared with NHEJ, this increases the challenge for gene editing.

NONHOMOLOGOUS END JOINING-BASED GENE EDITING FOR DUCHENNE MUSCULAR DYSTROPHY

Given the higher efficiency of NHEJ, there have been more efforts aimed at exploiting this approach where small deletions may be useful to provide partial correction. For example, for Duchenne muscular dystrophy (DMD), an X-linked recessive disorder that affects both heart and skeletal muscle, gene editing generates additional deletions that restore the reading frame, resulting in internal truncated but functional proteins. Dystrophin, the protein product of the DMD gene, is a large internally repetitive protein composed of 24 spectrin repeats throughout its midsection.[26,27] The DMD gene itself spans 2.5 M base pairs and includes 79 coding exons. Deletions that disrupt the reading frame ablate expression of the dystrophin protein, leading to DMD. Approximately 80% of DMD mutations are large mutations that span large intervals of thousands of base pairs, and most of these are deletions.[28] In contrast, in-frame deletions typically

lead to dystrophin protein production, which can be detected by immunoblotting or immunofluorescence detection using antidystrophin antibodies. In-frame deletions affect both the stability and function of dystrophin. For example, the middle portion of dystrophin has been implicated in binding nitric oxide synthase, which is important for regulating vascular tone and blood flow to muscle.[29] Nonetheless, restoring dystrophin's reading frame converts DMD to the milder Becker muscular dystrophy (BMD). However, BMD has an associated cardiomyopathy, and a detailed analysis of BMD-associated mutations found that onset of cardiomyopathy was earliest for mutations disrupting the amino-terminal actin-binding domain. BMD patients with mutations in spectrin repeats 17 to 19 had an intermediate age of cardiomyopathy onset, while those with mutations disrupting the third hinge and spectrin repeats 20 and 21 had the latest onset of cardiomyopathy.[30] These findings suggest that different domains may be more critical for some aspects of cardiac function compared with domains needed to rescue skeletal muscle function.

A detailed understanding of dystrophin's domain function is important, as CRISPR/Cas9 can be deployed to create new dystrophin gene deletions with the goal of restoring the reading frame. Approximately 13% of DMD patients have mutations in exons 48 to 50, resulting in loss of dystrophin.[31] Gene editing is designed to target exon 51 by generating deletions that disrupt the splicing inclusion sequences in exon 51, which then restores the reading frame and converts a DMD mutation into a BMD mutation (**Fig. 2**). This

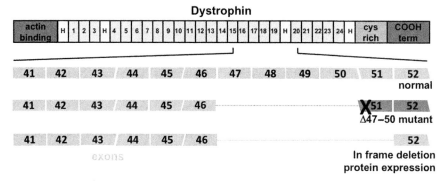

Fig. 2. CRISPR/Cas9 strategy for restoring the reading frame due to deletion mutations in the dystrophin gene. Deletions in the dystrophin gene disrupt the reading frame in DMD, and deletions of exons 47, 48, 49, and 50 affect 13% of DMD patients. Dystrophin is a large protein with an actin-binding domain at its amino terminus. There are 4 hinge (H) domains and 24 spectrin repeats that comprise the middle portion of the protein. The cysteine-rich (cys rich) region is needed for dystrophin function. The carboxy-terminal (COOH term) domain is dispensable. Guide RNAs directed toward splicing regulatory sequences in exon 51 (marked with an X) can be used to exclude this exon in the mRNA, which then results in exon 46 joining to exon 52. This restores the dystrophin reading frame, creating an internally truncated, but functional dystrophin protein. Similar strategies can be used to restore the reading frame in other regions of dystrophin.

rationale also underlies the antisense oligonucleotide (AON) drug eteplirsen.[32] AON-based therapies require repeated weekly intravenous dosing for DMD. Gene editing, if successful, in principle, should require only a single application.[33]

Preclinical studies in mice have documented the success of systemic gene editing to restore dystrophin expression in the *mdx* model of DMD.[34–38] Virally mediated systemic delivery of Cas9 and guide RNAs also corrected the dystrophin gene in the heart, resulting in dystrophin protein expression.[34,36,38,39] Several features make systemic in vivo genetic correction of DMD appealing. First, DMD as a severe disease has a greater risk-benefit ratio that milder disorders. Second, the X-linked recessive inheritance of DMD necessitates the correction of only the single X-chromosome. Lastly, NHEJ, rather than HDR, increases the feasibility of success. The drawbacks of applying CRISPR/Cas9 in human DMD are the limited data on safety of this approach and the need to conduct this using widespread viral delivery in children. Gene editing in DMD, by design, will also result in cardiac gene editing, and therefore may become the first use of gene editing in the human heart.

ANTISENSE OLIGONUCLEOTIDE-BASED GENETIC CORRECTION FOR DMD

Antisense oligonucleotide (AON)-based therapy is an alternative genetic corrective strategy that aims to manipulate RNA, rather than DNA. Eteplirsen is an AON drug that targets exon 51 of the DMD gene. As an AON, eteplirsen contains complementary sequences that hybridize to the RNA prior to splicing, and promotes exon exclusion from the mature mRNA.[32] This approach is conceptually similar to gene editing for its end effect, but does so by engaging RNA. In addition to US Food and Drug Administration approval of eteplirsen, the AON drug nusinersen was recently approved for the treatment of the autosomal-recessive spinal muscular atrophy, a neuromuscular disorder that affects young children.[40,41] AONs rely on chemical modifications of oligonucleotides, and these chemical modifications prolong drug half-life by avoiding endogenous nucleases that cleave double-stranded nucleic acid moieties.[42]

ANTISENSE OLIGONUCLEOTIDE APPLICATION FOR OTHER DISORDERS

Several other disorders with systemic features, including neuromuscular disease, have also been identified for application of AON therapy including limb girdle muscular dystrophy type 2C (LGMD 2C).[43] LGMD 2C is an autosomal-recessive disorder caused by loss of function mutations in *SCGC*, which encodes γ-sarcoglycan, a dystrophin-associated protein. LGMD 2C has similar findings to DMD, including progressive skeletal muscle wasting and weakness, along with cardiomyopathy.[44] In this case, AON-directed therapy is designed to promote retention of exons 4, 5, 6, and 7 from this 8-exon gene, which would remove nearly half the final protein product. This product, termed mini-gamma, was shown to be partially protective in animal models of LGMD 2C.

Mutations in the *LMNA* gene lead to various disorders, including cardiomyopathy. One disorder, Hutchinson Gulford Progeria, arises from a mutation that alters splicing and promotes the production of prelamin A, which is thought to underlie the toxicity related to this premature aging disorder. An AON-based approach has been tested in human cells and has demonstrated the capacity to alter production of prelamin A, which should be therapeutic for this disease.[45,46] Other approaches manipulating *LMNA* splicing using ASOs have also been developed.[47]

Autosomal-dominant *MYBPC3* mutations lead to HCM.[48] Using a mouse model of *Mybpc* mutations, it was shown that AON-induced exon skipping could produce an alternative transcript that restored protein expression and cardiac function.[49] Moreover, additional studies of *MYBPC3* suggests that trans-splicing events can happen, where splicing between two independent RNAs takes place.[50] In this case, splicing between the mutant and normal alleles could be used to bypass a specific mutation. However, at present the efficiency of trans-splicing is low and would need to be significantly augmented to have therapeutic benefit. These studies and others underlie the complexity of RNA splicing, which may be even more complicated in cardiomyopathy, as heart failure itself leads to alternative splicing patterns. For example, *TTN* truncating mutations are a common cause of DCM, and exon skipping has been tested for 3′ end *TTN* mutations.[51] In theory, it may be possible to use AON-directed strategies to reframe more *TTN* truncations, but the sheer size and complexity of *TTN* makes this task daunting.[52]

RNA-BASED GENE EDITING FOR MICROSATELLITE REPEAT EXPANSION DISORDERS

Recently, CRISPR/Cas9 has been directed against microsatellite repeat expansion disorders including myotonic dystrophy type 1 and 2.[53] Microsatellites are small units of repetitive DNA sequences. Expansion of these microsatellite repeats, typically on a single allele, is sufficient to cause disease; both myotonic dystrophy type 1 and 2 are associated with arrhythmias and cardiomyopathy.[54,55] In myotonic dystrophy type 1, the CTG trinucleotide in the *DMPK* gene on one allele expands to greater than 70 copies. Myotonic dystrophy type 2 arises from expansion of the CCTG repeat within the *CNBP/ZNF9* gene, in which the tetranucleotide repeat expands to many thousands of copies. These repeat expansions themselves have been the target of ASO-based treatment, and CRISPR/Cas9 has been engineered to recognize these repeats when expressed as RNA.[56]

MUTATION-INDEPENDENT GENETIC CORRECTION FOR HEART FAILURE

In each of the previously discussed strategies, genetic correction was directed at mutations directly responsible for disease. In applying this to human cardiomyopathy, many different, site-specific corrective strategies must be designed and tested. This feat is challenging from a clinical trial and regulatory perspective. Each AON or guide RNA would be useful for a very small number of individuals, which makes placebo-controlled trials, the regulatory standard, nearly impossible. This has prompted some to evaluate the possibility of broader genetic corrective avenues that would target normal genes in order to boost cardiac function. For example, gene therapy to upregulate SERCA was tested in heart failure with reduced ejection fraction.[57,58] Reducing phospholamban, even partially, may upregulate SERCA activity and thereby modulate Ca^{2+} mishandling that underlies heart failure.[59] It may be possible to use AON or gene editing to upregulate specific splice forms of sarcomere proteins that increase actomyosin interactions, and in effect make the heart more energetically efficient.

ETHICAL CONSIDERATIONS OF GENE EDITING

Gene editing is a powerful technique, and its application to the human genome has raised ethical questions owing to the capacity to alter the human germ line and therefore future generations.[60,61] Somatic correction of mutations or manipulation of a normal gene with the goal of treatment is distinct from germline correction (**Fig. 3**). Most recently, the capacity for germline correction was demonstrated when a fertilized oocyte carrying an *MYBPC3* allele was corrected using HDR gene editing.[62] Remarkably, the authors found the mutation correction rate was reasonably efficient in fertilized eggs, including template and nontemplate-directed HDR. The corrected zygotes were not implanted. However, it should be

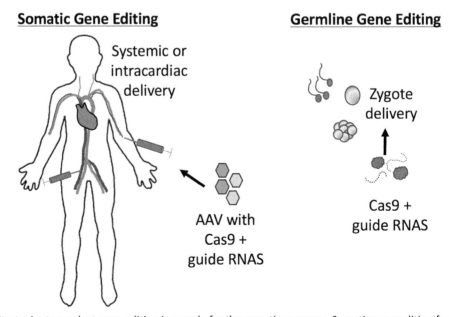

Fig. 3. Strategies to conduct gene editing in people for therapeutic purposes. Somatic gene editing for heart failure is expected to use adeno-associated virus (AAV) to deliver Cas9 and guide RNAs to the heart. This can be used for either systemic or intracardiac delivery. Germline gene editing delivers Cas9 protein and guide RNAs to a zygote to correct genetic mutations that cause disease. Cas9 can also be delivered directly into fertilized eggs using RNA encoding Cas9.

emphasized that the first step to collect and identify eggs relied on preimplantation genetic diagnosis (PGD) to define which zygotes carried the MYBPC3 mutation and which did not. As an autosomal-dominant disorder, 50% of the zygotes were mutation free simply by inheriting the nonmutant allele. These mutation-free zygotes can be implanted, as is routinely accomplished with PGD. PGD does not require gene editing, thus avoiding off-target mutations.[63]

HOMOLOGY-DIRECTED REPAIR IN NONDIVIDING CARDIOMYOCYTES

The degree to which cardiomyocytes can complete HDR has been debated. In principle, HDR is thought to require a round of cellular replication. Because nearly all cardiomyocytes are postmitotic, this would suggest that HDR could only be used to address dividing cells in the heart. However, gene editing in skeletal myofibers, which are terminally differentiated, was achieved using HDR.[38] Notably these studies used a Cas9 expressed under the control of a modified muscle creatine kinase promoter active only in mature myofibers and inactive in muscle stem cells. More recently, several studies have shown HDR in postnatal mouse hearts, indicating that HDR may not require cell replication[64,65] and suggesting that genetic correction of site specific mutations may be more feasible than predicted.

DELIVERING GENE EDITING MACHINERY TO THE HEART

Viral vectors are the primary delivery modality for Cas9. Specifically, adeno-associated virus (AAV) is a preferred virus, because specific strains display high tropism for cardiomyocytes.[66] The major limitation of AAV is its small cargo capacity. As noted previously, certain Cas9s fit more readily within the carrying capacity of AAV. However, even SaCas9 has reached its limit with AAV, necessitating second viruses to carry the guide RNAs.[67] With viral delivery, it may be necessary to terminate Cas9 activity either through guides that target the Cas9 gene or through drug-regulatable domains that target Cas9 for proteolytically digestion.[17] Immunity is known to develop against AAV capsids, and Cas9 itself may be immunogenic. Although this characteristic could help limit its activity, it would also limit redelivery of Cas9.

FIDELITY OF GENE EDITING

Cas9 as a nuclease can produce unwanted off-target and on-target mutations. Off-target mutations are created at sites remote from the intended target. Estimating the frequency of off-target mutations for somatic gene correction requires detection of low-frequency events. Where gene editing is carried out on single cells that subsequently produce clonal expansion of the corrected cell, it is possible to conduct whole-genome or whole-exome sequencing to assess off-target mutations. However, in applying gene editing to the heart, the off-target mutations may differ from cell to cell and would not be detected by even whole-genome sequencing. Estimating off-target mutations in zygotes has been done in genetically engineered mice, but this too is complicated by the rate of new mutations that occurs in every zygote.[68]

In addition to off-target mutations, NHEJ produces a range of deletions, rather than single events. Deep sequencing across these sites can be used to estimate the fidelity of on-target events. From studies in the *mdx* mouse, it appears that only a small population of properly corrected cells can produce a greater percentage of corrected mRNA species.[38,39,69] Ultimately, a relatively small percentage of corrected cells produces a higher-than-expected amount of dystrophin protein. This may relate to the selective advantage of corrected cells over uncorrected cells, as uncorrected cells may be more prone to injury and necrosis.

FUTURE CONSIDERATIONS

The advent of gene editing has already made a significant impact in the laboratory setting, where it is now routinely used to make highly useful models of disease or to demonstrate the feasibility of gene correction. Transitioning this laboratory-based tool to *in vivo* human gene editing for the treatment of heart failure is on the horizon, but will require evidence that this process is both safe and efficacious. The cardiac tropism of AAV as a delivery vehicle, and the ability to use catheter-based approaches to introduce AAVs carrying Cas9 and guide RNAs into the heart, make it an attractive target for gene editing.

REFERENCES

1. Collins FS, Morgan M, Patrinos A. The human genome project: lessons from large scale biology. Science 2003;300(5617):286–9.
2. Karczewski KJ, Weisburd B, Thomas B, et al. The ExAC browser: displaying reference data information from over 60 000 exomes. Nucleic Acids Res 2017;45(D1):D840–d845.

3. Lek M, Karczewski KJ, Minikel EV, et al. Analysis of protein-coding genetic variation in 60,706 humans. Nature 2016;536(7616):285–91.

4. Gaj T, Gersbach CA, Barbas CF 3rd. ZFN, TALEN, and CRISPR/Cas-based methods for genome engineering. Trends Biotechnol 2013;31(7):397–405.

5. Urnov FD, Miller JC, Lee Y, et al. Highly efficient endogenous human gene correction using designed zinc-finger nucleases. Nature 2005; 435(7042):646–51.

6. Cermak T, Doyle EL, Christian M, et al. Efficient design and assembly of custom TALEN and other TAL effector-based constructs for DNA targeting. Nucleic Acids Res 2011;39(12):e82.

7. Christian M, Cermak T, Doyle EL, et al. Targeting DNA double-strand breaks with TAL effector nucleases. Genetics 2010;186(2):757–61.

8. Lei Y, Guo X, Liu Y, et al. Efficient targeted gene disruption in Xenopus embryos using engineered transcription activator-like effector nucleases (TALENs). Proc Natl Acad Sci U S A 2012;109(43): 17484–9.

9. He Z, Proudfoot C, Whitelaw BA, et al. Comparison of CRISPR/Cas9 and TALENS on editing an integrated EGFP gene in the genome of HEK293FT cells. Springerplus 2016;5(1):814.

10. Gupta RM, Musunuru K. Expanding the genetic editing tool kit: ZFNs, TALENs, and CRISPR-Cas9. J Clin Invest 2014;124(10):4154–61.

11. Doetschman T, Georgieva T. Gene editing with CRISPR/Cas9 RNA-directed nuclease. Circ Res 2017;120(5):876–94.

12. Jinek M, Chylinski K, Fonfara I, et al. A programmable dual-RNA-guided DNA endonuclease in adaptive bacterial immunity. Science 2012;337(6096):816–21.

13. Cong L, Ran FA, Cox D, et al. Multiplex genome engineering using CRISPR/Cas systems. Science 2013;339(6121):819–23.

14. Ran FA, Hsu PD, Wright J, et al. Genome engineering using the CRISPR-Cas9 system. Nat Protoc 2013;8(11):2281–308.

15. Wu X, Scott DA, Kriz AJ, et al. Genome-wide binding of the CRISPR endonuclease Cas9 in mammalian cells. Nat Biotechnol 2014;32(7):670–6.

16. Cho SW, Kim S, Kim Y, et al. Analysis of off-target effects of CRISPR/Cas-derived RNA-guided endonucleases and nickases. Genome Res 2014;24(1): 132–41.

17. Maji B, Moore CL, Zetsche B, et al. Multidimensional chemical control of CRISPR-Cas9. Nat Chem Biol 2017;13(1):9–11.

18. Fonfara I, Le Rhun A, Chylinski K, et al. Phylogeny of Cas9 determines functional exchangeability of dual-RNA and Cas9 among orthologous type II CRISPR-Cas systems. Nucleic Acids Res 2014; 42(4):2577–90.

19. Ran FA, Cong L, Yan WX, et al. In vivo genome editing using Staphylococcus aureus Cas9. Nature 2015;520(7546):186–91.

20. Hou Z, Zhang Y, Propson NE, et al. Efficient genome engineering in human pluripotent stem cells using Cas9 from Neisseria meningitidis. Proc Natl Acad Sci U S A 2013;110(39):15644–9.

21. Tycho J, Myer VE, Hsu PD. Methods for optimizing CRISPR-Cas9 genome editing specificity. Mol Cell 2017;63(3):355–70.

22. Wang X, Huang X, Fang X, et al. CRISPR-Cas9 system as a versatile tool for genome engineering in human cells. Mol Ther Nucleic Acids 2016; 5(11):e388.

23. Marian AJ, Braunwald E. Hypertrophic cardiomyopathy: genetics, pathogenesis, clinical manifestations, diagnosis, and therapy. Circ Res 2017; 121(7):749–70.

24. McNally EM, Mestroni L. Dilated cardiomyopathy: genetic determinants and mechanisms. Circ Res 2017;121(7):731–48.

25. McNally E, MacLeod H, Dellefave-Castillo L. Arrhythmogenic right ventricular cardiomyopathy. In: Adam MP, Ardinger HH, Pagon RA, et al, editors. GeneReviews(R). Seattle (WA): University of Washington, Seattle; 1993.

26. Gao QQ, McNally EM. The dystrophin complex: structure, function, and implications for therapy. Compr Physiol 2015;5(3):1223–39.

27. Kamdar F, Garry DJ. Dystrophin-deficient cardiomyopathy. J Am Coll Cardiol 2016;67(21):2533–46.

28. Bladen CL, Salgado D, Monges S, et al. The TREAT-NMD DMD global database: analysis of more than 7,000 Duchenne muscular dystrophy mutations. Hum Mutat 2015;36(4):395–402.

29. Lai Y, Thomas GD, Yue Y, et al. Dystrophins carrying spectrin-like repeats 16 and 17 anchor nNOS to the sarcolemma and enhance exercise performance in a mouse model of muscular dystrophy. J Clin Invest 2009;119(3):624–35.

30. Kaspar RW, Allen HD, Ray WC, et al. Analysis of dystrophin deletion mutations predicts age of cardiomyopathy onset in Becker muscular dystrophy. Circ Cardiovasc Genet 2009;2(6):544–51.

31. Aartsma-Rus A, Fokkema I, Verschuuren J, et al. Theoretic applicability of antisense-mediated exon skipping for Duchenne muscular dystrophy mutations. Hum Mutat 2009;30(3):293–9.

32. Aartsma-Rus A, Straub V, Hemmings R, et al. Development of exon skipping therapies for Duchenne muscular dystrophy: a critical review and a perspective on the outstanding issues. Nucleic Acid Ther 2017;27(5):251–9.

33. Calos MP. The CRISPR way to think about Duchenne's. N Engl J Med 2016;374(17):1684–6.

34. Long C, Amoasii L, Mireault AA, et al. Postnatal genome editing partially restores dystrophin

expression in a mouse model of muscular dystrophy. Science 2016;351(6271):400–3.

35. Long C, McAnally JR, Shelton JM, et al. Prevention of muscular dystrophy in mice by CRISPR/Cas9-mediated editing of germline DNA. Science 2014; 345(6201):1184–8.

36. Nelson CE, Hakim CH, Ousterout DG, et al. In vivo genome editing improves muscle function in a mouse model of Duchenne muscular dystrophy. Science 2016;351(6271):403–7.

37. Tabebordbar M, Zhu K, Cheng JKW, et al. In vivo gene editing in dystrophic mouse muscle and muscle stem cells. Science 2016;351(6271):407–11.

38. Bengtsson NE, Hall JK, Odom GL, et al. Muscle-specific CRISPR/Cas9 dystrophin gene editing ameliorates pathophysiology in a mouse model for Duchenne muscular dystrophy. Nat Commun 2017; 8:14454.

39. El Refaey M, Xu L, Gao Y, et al. vivo genome editing restores dystrophin expression and cardiac function in dystrophic mice. Circ Res 2017;121(8):923–9.

40. Corey DR. Nusinersen, an antisense oligonucleotide drug for spinal muscular atrophy. Nat Neurosci 2017;20(4):497–9.

41. Finkel RS, Chiriboga CA, Vajsar J, et al. Treatment of infantile-onset spinal muscular atrophy with nusinersen: a phase 2, open-label, dose-escalation study. Lancet 2016;388(10063):3017–26.

42. Khvorova A, Watts JK. The chemical evolution of oligonucleotide therapies of clinical utility. Nat Biotechnol 2017;35(3):238–48.

43. Gao QQ, Wyatt E, Goldstein JA, et al. Reengineering a transmembrane protein to treat muscular dystrophy using exon skipping. J Clin Invest 2015; 125(11):4186–95.

44. Narayanaswami P, Weiss M, Selcen D, et al. Evidence-based guideline summary: diagnosis and treatment of limb-girdle and distal dystrophies: report of the guideline development subcommittee of the American Academy of Neurology and the practice issues review panel of the American Association of Neuromuscular & Electrodiagnostic Medicine. Neurology 2014;83(16):1453–63.

45. Lee JM, Nobumori C, Tu Y, et al. Modulation of LMNA splicing as a strategy to treat prelamin A diseases. J Clin Invest 2016;126(4):1592–602.

46. Harhouri K, Navarro C, Baquerre C, et al. Antisense-based progerin downregulation in HGPS-like patients' cells. Cells 2016;5(3) [pii:E31].

47. Scharner J, Figeac N, Ellis JA, et al. Ameliorating pathogenesis by removing an exon containing a missense mutation: a potential exon-skipping therapy for laminopathies. Gene Ther 2015;22(6): 503–15.

48. Alfares AA, Kelly MA, McDermott G, et al. Results of clinical genetic testing of 2,912 probands with hypertrophic cardiomyopathy: expanded panels offer limited additional sensitivity. Genet Med 2015; 17(11):880–8.

49. Gedicke-Hornung C, Behrens-Gawlik V, Reischmann S, et al. Rescue of cardiomyopathy through U7snRNA-mediated exon skipping in Mybpc3-targeted knock-in mice. EMBO Mol Med 2013;5(7):1128–45.

50. Prondzynski M, Kramer E, Laufer SD, et al. Evaluation of MYBPC3 trans-splicing and gene replacement as therapeutic options in human iPSC-derived cardiomyocytes. Mol Ther Nucleic Acids 2017;7:475–86.

51. Gramlich M, Pane LS, Zhou Q, et al. Antisense-mediated exon skipping: a therapeutic strategy for titin-based dilated cardiomyopathy. EMBO Mol Med 2015;7(5):562–76.

52. Roberts AM, Ware JS, Herman DS, et al. Integrated allelic, transcriptional, and phenomic dissection of the cardiac effects of titin truncations in health and disease. Sci Transl Med 2015;7(270): 270ra6.

53. Batra R, Nelles DA, Pirie E, et al. Elimination of toxic microsatellite repeat expansion RNA by RNA-targeting Cas9. Cell 2017;170(5):899–912.e10.

54. Chong-Nguyen C, Wahbi K, Algalarrondo V, et al. Association between mutation size and cardiac involvement in myotonic dystrophy type 1: an analysis of the DM1-heart registry. Circ Cardiovasc Genet 2017;10(3) [pii:e001526].

55. Groh WJ. Arrhythmias in the muscular dystrophies. Heart Rhythm 2012;9(11):1890–5.

56. Thornton CA, Wang E, Carrell EM. Myotonic dystrophy: approach to therapy. Curr Opin Genet Dev 2017;44:135–40.

57. Hulot JS, Salem JE, Redheuil A, et al. Effect of intracoronary administration of AAV1/SERCA2a on ventricular remodelling in patients with advanced systolic heart failure: results from the AGENT-HF randomized phase 2 trial. Eur J Heart Fail 2017;19(11): 1534–41.

58. Jessup M, Greenberg B, Mancini D, et al. Calcium upregulation by percutaneous administration of gene therapy in cardiac disease (CUPID): a phase 2 trial of intracoronary gene therapy of sarcoplasmic reticulum Ca2+-ATPase in patients with advanced heart failure. Circulation 2011;124(3):304–13.

59. Kaneko M, Hashikami K, Yamamoto S, et al. Phospholamban ablation using CRISPR/Cas9 system improves mortality in a murine heart failure model. PLoS One 2016;11(12):e0168486.

60. Ormond KE, Mortlock DP, Scholes DT, et al. Human germline genome editing. Am J Hum Genet 2017; 101(2):167–76.

61. Pei D, Beier DW, Levy-Lahad E, et al. Human embryo editing: opportunities and importance of transnational cooperation. Cell Stem Cell 2017;21(4): 423–6.

62. Ma H, Marti-Gutierrez N, Park SW, et al. Correction of a pathogenic gene mutation in human embryos. Nature 2017;548(7668):413–9.

63. Brezina PR, Kutteh WH. Clinical applications of pre-implantation genetic testing. BMJ 2015;350:g7611.

64. Ishizu T, Higo S, Masumura Y, et al. Targeted genome replacement via homology-directed repair in non-dividing cardiomyocytes. Sci Rep 2017; 7(1):9363.

65. Xie C, Zhang YP, Song L, et al. Genome editing with CRISPR/Cas9 in postnatal mice corrects PRKAG2 cardiac syndrome. Cell Res 2016;26(10):1099–111.

66. VanDusen NJ, Guo Y, Gu W, et al. CASAAV: a CRISPR-based platform for rapid dissection of gene function in vivo. Curr Protoc Mol Biol 2017; 120. 31.11.31-31.11.14.

67. Friedland AE, Baral R, Singhal P, et al. Characterization of Staphylococcus aureus Cas9: a smaller Cas9 for all-in-one adeno-associated virus delivery and paired nickase applications. Genome Biol 2015;16:257.

68. Schaefer KA, Wu WH, Colgan DF, et al. Unexpected mutations after CRISPR-Cas9 editing in vivo. Nat Methods 2017;14(6):547–8.

69. Zhang Y, Long C, Li H, et al. CRISPR-Cpf1 correction of muscular dystrophy mutations in human cardiomyocytes and mice. Sci Adv 2017;3(4): e1602814.

Controversies Surrounding Exercise in Genetic Cardiomyopathies

Gourg Atteya, MD, Rachel Lampert, MD*

KEYWORDS

- Genetic cardiomyopathies • Sudden cardiac death • Exercise

KEY POINTS

- Exercise has established health benefits among all age groups, both physical and psychological.
- Patients with genetic cardiomyopathies are at risk of sudden cardiac death; to what extent exercise increases risk is controversial.
- Patients with arrhythmogenic right ventricular cardiomyopathy who exercise vigorously, particularly endurance exercise, seem to have a heightened risk for progression of disease, as well as ventricular arrhythmia. Exact levels of exercise that are safe have not been defined; however, the American Heart Association minimum recommendation seems to be safe in this group.
- Risk of vigorous exercise for patients with hypertrophic cardiomyopathy is unclear. Recent evidence showed moderate exercise to be associated with better exercise capacity and no signal of adverse cardiac remodeling or arrhythmias.
- Patients with dilated cardiomyopathy have little evidence to support or recommend against exercise; however, safety seems evident with low-intensity exercise such as cardiac rehabilitation.

EPIDEMIOLOGY OF SUDDEN CARDIAC DEATH IN ATHLETES

Whether athletes have higher incidences of sudden cardiac death (SCD) than nonathletes is an active area of research, as is understanding the underlying etiologies of SCD in the athlete. In population-based studies, incidence of sudden death in young people under 35 is reported from 1.3 to 2.8 per 100,000 person-years.[1–4] Some studies suggest that athletes have a higher rate of SCD than nonathletes. In a prospective study of more than 2000 high schools, the overall incidence of sudden death was 0.63 per 100,000, whereas incidence of SCD in student athletes (excluding commotion cordis) was 0.95 per 100,000,[5] translating to a 3.65 relative risk of SCD for athletes. The US National Registry of Sudden Death in Athletes, which collected cases about SCD from media reports and other sources for more than 30 years, reported an average of 66 deaths per year that was calculated, using an estimated denominator of 10.7 million participants in sports per year, to an incidence of SCD in athletes of 0.61 per 100,000 person-years.[6] However, media reports may underestimate SCD incidence in athletes. In a Danish study, incidence of SCD was not different between noncompetitive and competitive athletes, with increased incidence of SCD in those ages 36 to 49 years; however, the general population had a higher incidence compared with all athlete groups.[7] Also, in a recent Canadian study, the incidence of SCD was 0.76 cases per 100,000 athlete-years, with no

Disclosure statement: Dr. Lampert: Medtronic, Advisory Board and research grant, Abbott, research grant.
Department of Internal Medicine/Cardiology, Yale School of Medicine, 789 Howard Avenue, New Haven, CT 06520, USA
* Corresponding author. Section of Cardiology, Yale School of Medicine, New Haven, CT 06520.
E-mail address: Rachel.lampert@yale.edu

Heart Failure Clin 14 (2018) 189–200
https://doi.org/10.1016/j.hfc.2017.12.008
1551-7136/18/© 2018 Elsevier Inc. All rights reserved.

significant difference between competitive and noncompetitive sports participants.[8] In National Collegiate Athletic Association (NCAA) athletes[9] there was an overall incidence of SCD in NCAA athletes of 2.3 per 100,000 athlete-years.

The exact breakdown of etiologic factors of SCD in athletes remains controversial. In the early series from the US National Registry of Sudden Death in Athletes, more than one-third of cases were found to be due to hypertrophic cardiomyopathy (HCM).[6] In Italy, arrhythmogenic right ventricular cardiomyopathy (ARVC) was reported as the most common cause of SCD in a postmortem study of 60 persons who died suddenly.[10] More recent series have found that autopsy-negative (structurally normal heart) cases represent the most common cause of sudden death in athletes,[9,11] as well as young people in general,[2–4] with HCM accounting for less than 10%[9,11] (**Fig. 1**). There are obvious differences in ascertainment methodology, as well as potential reporting

biases in voluntary registries, which may explain some of the differences between study results. Understanding the role that genetic cardiomyopathies may play in the sudden death of athletes or of young people during exercise, remains an important avenue of research.

EXERCISE AS A TRIGGER

To what extent exertion triggers SCD in the general population is also controversial. Initial reports from the US National Registry of Sudden Death in Athletes suggested that more than 80% of the deaths occurred during competition or training.[6] However, several recent population-based studies showed about half of SCD occurred either during sleep or at rest,[2,4] with just 11% occurring during exertion.[4] Postmortem-based studies have also found about half of sudden deaths in the young occur during rest or sleep.[8] Among athletes in the NCAA, 56% of SCD

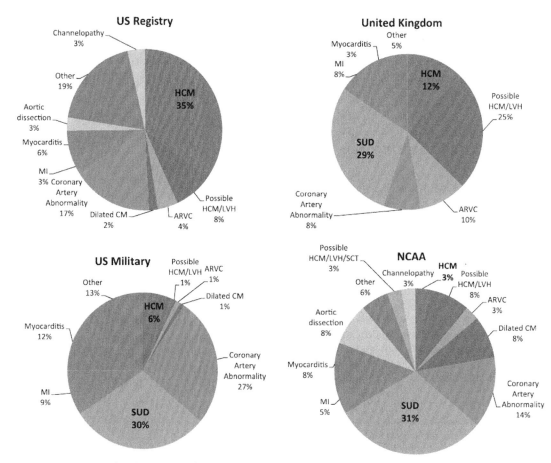

Fig. 1. Comparison of pathogenesis of SCD in US registry, UK, US military, and the NCAA. CM, cardiomyopathy; LVH, left ventricular hypotrophy, MI, myocardial infarction; SCT, sickle cell trait; SUD, sudden unexplained death. (*From* Harmon KG, Drezner JA, Maleszewski JJ, et al. Pathogenesis of sudden cardiac death in National Collegiate Athletic Association athletes. Circ Arrhythm and Electrophysiol. 2014;7:202; with permission.)

occurred with exertion.[12,13] In a prospective study investigating the incidence of SCD in all high school students occurring on school campus, 26 students died suddenly, with 69% in athletes and all during exercise.[5] An important limitation is the small number of cases, with no clear histopathologic diagnosis. Among older individuals, sports-associated SCD in the middle-aged population represented just 5% of all SCD cases (63 out of total 1247 SCD).[14]

Associations of ventricular arrhythmia with exercise were examined in the implantable cardioverter-defibrillator (ICD) Sports Safety Registry, which followed athletes with ICDs who engaged in vigorous and competitive sports. In that study, more appropriate shocks for ventricular arrhythmias occurred while patients were active; however, there was no difference between competition and other physical activity.[15] Differences in methodology of these studies, ranging from voluntary-reporting registries (eg, the US National Registry of Sudden Death in Athletes), to population-based studies, to postmortem-based studies, as well as differences in populations, may explain the wide variation in these data.

HEALTH BENEFITS OF EXERCISE

The health benefits of exercise have been studied extensively, and exercise has been promoted in the United States as a national public health agenda for all ages for many years.[16–19]

The cardiovascular health benefits of an active lifestyle are well-established.[20,21] Both men and women with reported increased levels of physical activity and fitness have remarkable reductions in relative risk of death (by about 20%–35%).[22–25] Both baseline fitness and increase in physical fitness are related to better outcomes (**Fig. 2**). In addition to longevity,[26–28] increasing levels of activity are associated with decreased incidence of coronary artery disease[26,29] and diabetes.[30] This may be due in part to improvements in lipid[31] and glucose levels.[32] In a recent prospective population-based study, physical activity was inversely associated with risk of cardiovascular disease, especially among those aged 65 years and older.[33] Risks of a sedentary life in children and adolescents include higher risk of obesity, diabetes, hypertension, and even cancer.[18,34–36] In a European study of 1500 adolescents, those who consumed a healthy diet and were active had better cardiovascular risk scores[37] (**Fig. 3**).

The benefits of physical activity extend beyond just physical health to mental and social health and quality of life. Exercise increases quality of life in adults[38] and adolescents,[39] as well as perceived health.[40] Those benefits are evident across all age groups. In children; sedentary lifestyle was associated with higher rates of depression and fatigue.[41–43] In a recent systematic review of adolescents, screen time of more than 2 to 3 hours per day led to worse mental health

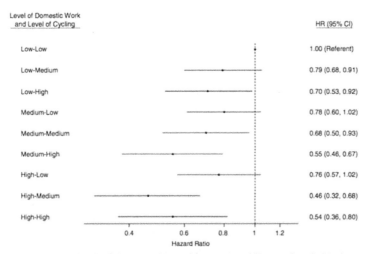

Fig. 2. Level of physical activity and risk of coronary heart disease in middle-aged and elderly persons. Hazard ratios and 95% confidence intervals of coronary heart disease for the combined domestic work and cycling variable in multi-variable model 2, Rotterrdam Study, 1997–2012. In every combination, the tertile of domestic work is mentioned first and cycling second. Model 2 is adjusted for age, sex, and other physical activity types, smoking, alcohol consumption, diet, and education. Circles indicate hazard ratios; horizontal lines indicate 95% confidence intervals. CI, confidence interval; HR, hazard ratio. (*From* Koolhaas CM, Dhana K, Golubic R, et al. Physical activity types and coronary heart disease risk in middle-aged and elderly persons: The Rotterdam Study. Am J Epidemiol. 2016;183(8):735; with permission.)

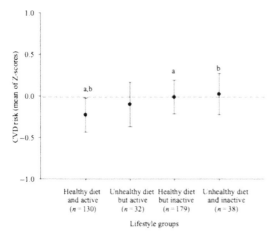

Fig. 3. Active lifestyle and healthy diet and CVD risk scores in adolescents. (*From* Cuenca-Garcia M, Ortega FB, Ruiz JR, et al. Combined influence of healthy diet and active lifestyle on cardiovascular disease risk factors in adolescents. Scand J Med Sci Sports 2014;24(3):557; with permission.)

outcomes.[44] In a systematic review of more than 50 studies, there was a positive association between physical activity and academic performance, academic behavior, and cognitive skills and attitudes.[45] Another review showed physical activity as the most published and consistent variable with positive impact on student's academic achievement.[46] For the elderly, regular physical activity has consistently proven effective in preventing or delaying physical and cognitive disabilities,[47–49] as well as improving depressive symptoms, quality of life, and self-esteem.[50,51]

Based on these extensive data regarding exercise benefits, current clinical guidelines for prevention of cardiovascular disease recommend 150 minutes of moderate or greater intensity, or at least 60 to 75 minutes of vigorous exercise each week.[19,27,52]

EXERCISE IN SPECIFIC GENETIC CARDIOMYOPATHIES
Arrhythmogenic Right Ventricular Cardiomyopathy

Clinical, pathologic, and genetic features of ARVC are beyond the scope of this article. In general, overall mortality in ARVC ranges from 0.08% to 3.6% per year.[53] Initial reports, based on studies at tertiary referral centers, predominantly included high-risk patients and may have overestimated mortality, with recent studies of community-based patient cohorts showing more favorable long-term outcome for treated index patients and family members (annual mortality <1%).[54–56]

Evidence is mounting that endurance exercise may be detrimental in ARVC, with an increased risk of arrhythmias both acutely and chronically, as well as an increase in symptomatic progression of RV dysfunction. Acutely, exercise may trigger lethal arrhythmias, with an early multicenter series of 42 postmortem cases attributed to ARVC showed 34 deaths (81%) to be sudden in nature with almost half of these during exercise.[57] Similarly, 1 of the earliest studies from Italy describing SCD with ARVC found that 10 out of 12 subjects died during exercise.[10] In a study of athletes with ICDs, patients with ARVC were the most likely among the patient groups to experience ventricular arrhythmias and even required multiple shocks during sports participation or physical activity.[58]

In the long-term, exercise was noted to promote expression of the right ventricle (RV) dysfunction in ARVC, with endurance exercisers developing symptoms earlier in life than the sedentary. In the Johns Hopkins ARVC registry, 87 individuals with desmosomal mutations were evaluated in terms of their physical activity.[59] As shown in **Fig. 4**, endurance athletes were more likely to develop ventricular arrhythmias and heart failure over a mean follow-up of 8.4 years compared with the nonathletes. Also, 6 of 8 individuals in the top activity quartile who continued with significant exercise after their diagnosis experienced their first ventricular arrhythmia event during follow-up compared with only 1 of 8 individuals who reduced their exercise after diagnosis. A similar study of 108 index cases in the North American multidisciplinary study of ARVC classified patients as competitive, recreational, or inactive in terms of sports participation.[60] Over follow-up of 3 years, competitive athletes were diagnosed with ARVC at a younger age, and had twice the risk of the adverse events, mainly due to increased ventricular arrhythmias, with no significant difference between the inactive and recreational sports groups. Similarly, in a study of 37 PKP2 mutation carriers from 10 unrelated families, those participating in endurance and higher-intensity exercise had worse adverse outcomes.[61] Another study of 267 subjects showed again that participation in strenuous activity after the diagnosis of ARVC was associated with a higher burden of life-threatening arrhythmias at follow-up.[62]

Physiologic studies have suggested mechanisms through which exercise may exacerbate ARVC expression. Hemodynamically, exercise impacts the RV out of proportion to the left ventricle (LV). In athletes, RV shear stress increased 125% with prolonged strenuous exercise in comparison with 14% on the LV.[63] With such an increased stretch on the thin-walled RV, exercise in individuals with ARVC is thought to promote further

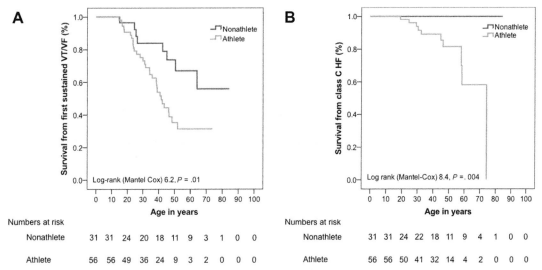

Fig. 4. Exercise impact on arrhythmia and heart failure in ARVC. (*A*) Cumulative lifetime survival free of sustained ventricular arrhythmias and (*B*) stage C heart failure stratified by participation in endurance athletics. Event-free survival from sustained arrhythmias and stage C heart failure is significantly lower among endurance athletes. HF, heart failure; VT/VF, ventricular tachycardia/ventricular fibrillation (sustained ventricular arrhythmia). (*From James CA, Bhonsale A, Tichnell C, et al. Exercise increases age-related penetrance and arrhythmic risk in arrhythmogenic right ventricular dysplasia/cardiomyopathy-associated desmosomal mutation carriers. J Am Coll Cardiol 2013;62(14):1294; with permission.*)

breakdown of the genetically abnormal desmosome, which might trigger fibrofatty replacement of the RV walls.

Experimental evidence also supports the detrimental effect of exercise in ARVC. In a heterozygous plakoglobin-deficient mouse model undergoing vigorous exercise, in comparison with wild-type control mice, the mutant mice demonstrated a propensity for developing features characteristic of the ARVC phenotype (RV enlargement, systolic dysfunction, and ventricular arrhythmias).[64]

How much exercise is safe in patients with arrhythmogenic right ventricular cardiomyopathy?

Based on many data showing the deleterious effects of vigorous exercise, both disease-based and athlete-based guidelines have recommended restriction of patients with ARVC from competitive or vigorous exercise. The 2015 American Heart Association (AHA) and American College of Cardiology (ACC) Eligibility and Disqualification Recommendation for Competitive Athletes gave a class III (not recommended) indication for patients with a definite, borderline, or even possible diagnosis of ARVC to participate in competitive sports, with the exception of low-intensity class 1A sports.[65] Similarly, the disease-based 2015 International Task Force Consensus Statement on Treatment of ARVC gave a class IIa recommendation for individuals with definite ARVC to refrain from any

athletic activities other than recreational low-intensity sports[53] and for asymptomatic genotype carriers without an ARVC phenotype to consider avoiding competitive sports.

In a study of *PKP2* mutation carriers, family members who restricted exercise at or below the AHA-recommended minimum threshold of a median exercise intensity of 450 to 750 minutes per week had more favorable outcomes with no sustained ventricular arrhythmias,[61] suggesting a more favorable outcome when unaffected desmosomal mutation carriers are restricted from endurance and high-intensity athletics but not from AHA-recommended levels of exercise (**Fig. 5**). In another study of nonfamilial ARVC cases, endurance exercise had a negative impact on RV structure and increased the prevalence of arrhythmias.[66] Although these studies suggested the effect was graded, with no safe level beyond the AHA recommendation, other studies have found that type of exercise may play a role. In a study of the North American multidisciplinary study of ARVC, competitive sports were associated with worse outcomes, whereas recreational activity was not.[60] To what degree patients with ARVC can exercise and enjoy all the attendant benefits remains an important avenue of research.

Hypertrophic Cardiomyopathy

Clinical, pathologic, and genetic features of HCM are beyond the scope of this article.

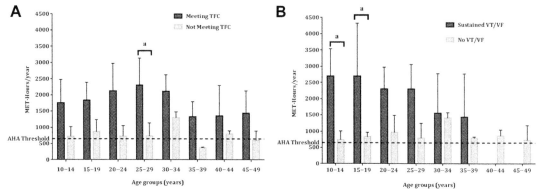

Fig. 5. (*A*) Median exercise intensity hours per year (MET-Hours/year) in metabolic equivalent hours before diagnosis in 5-year age increments compared with (*B*) the AHA-recommended minimum stratified by diagnosis by 2010 Task Force Criteria (TFC) and VT/VF history. The dotted black line represents the upper bound of the AHA-recommended minimum exercise (650). Error bars depict interquartile range. The asterisk denotes statistically significant *P*<.05. (*From* Sawant AC, Te Riele AS, Tichnell C, et al. Safety of American Heart Association-recommended minimum exercise for desmosomal mutation carriers. Heart Rhythm 2016;13(1):204.)

Exercise and sudden cardiac death in hypertrophic cardiomyopathy

In general, incidence of sudden death in HCM is highest in children and decreases into older adulthood. Initial data from tertiary referral centers reported incidence was up to 6% per year. However, recent data of 474 subjects aged 7 to 29 years, showed a much lower death rate of 0.54% per year. In that study, the rate of aborted life-threatening events, including ICD-treated ventricular arrhythmias, resuscitated arrest, or heart transplant, was close to 2% per year. This shows improving survival in this population is most likely due to current medical and device therapies.[67] For patients older than 60 years, even with conventional risk factors, incidence of mortality is low at 0.64% per year.[68]

The risk of SCD associated with exercise in individuals with HCM is a topic of ongoing research. How much exercise in these individuals is safe is not yet clear. As previously described, early retrospective studies suggested that HCM was responsible for a significant percentage of sudden death in athletes[6]; however, more contemporary studies show a much smaller contribution. For a patient with a known diagnosis of HCM, it is not known whether participation in vigorous or competitive exercise increases risk of SCD. Although the US National Registry of Sudden Death in Athletes suggested that death was more likely to occur during exercise, other studies have shown that most SCD events in HCM occur at rest, with only a small percentage occurring during or following exercise.[2,3,10]

In general, risk stratification for SCD in patients with HCM has improved over the last decade. Negative predictive value is good but not 100%

for those without markers of risk. Currently, there are 2 primary approaches to estimating SCD risk and other novel risk factors are emerging. In the United States, most recent ACC/AHA guidelines (2011), outline 4 primary clinical risk factors, any of which could prompt a recommendation for an ICD.[69] In Europe, the 2014 European Society of Cardiology guidelines take a different approach, which is designed to take into account the different effect size of individual risk factors and the continuous nature of risk factors such as LV wall thickness.[70]

For patients with HCM at risk high enough to warrant an ICD, there are now data suggesting that risks of vigorous, competitive exercise are low. In a series of athletes with ICDs who had chosen to compete, including 75 HCM subjects, there were no deaths or resuscitated arrests, or arrhythmia-related or shock-related injuries, related to sports.[15,58] These data are insufficient to describe the risk as zero; however, they do suggest the risk is low. The HCM subpopulation of this group is currently under further analysis to describe risk factors for arrhythmia recurrences in these athletes.

For those not risk at high enough for an ICD based on current risk prediction algorithms, the overall risk of SCD is low but not zero. Whether exercise would increase risk in these otherwise low-risk patients is unknown. In the series of athletes previously described who had died of HCM, the disease was diagnosed postmortem. Whether they would have met criteria for an ICD had the HCM been diagnosed previously is difficult to know. Management around sports and vigorous exercise is thus difficult for the HCM patient whose clinical characteristics do not suggest need for an ICD. Concerns related to SCD during exercise led to disease-specific guidelines on HCM from both the European Society for Cardiology (2014)[70] and the AHA (2011).[69] Sports-specific guidelines for eligibility for competitive sports from both Europe[71] and the United States[65] recommend against competitive sports participation in those patients.

Recommendations for participation in competitive athletics for asymptomatic, genotype-positive HCM patients without evidence of LV hypertrophy by 2-dimensional echocardiography and cardiac MRI vary. US guidelines endorse sports participation for this group, whereas European guidelines do not. There are no current data on the safety of sports for athletes who are genotype-positive but phenotype-negative for HCM.

Further research is warranted to further understanding of the short-term and long-term safety of exercise at moderate and higher levels of intensity. The Lifestyle and Exercise in Hypertrophic Cardiomyopathy (LIVE-HCM) study is enrolling subjects with HCM, as well as genotype-positive, phenotype-negative individuals, and following them prospectively to determine the risks versus safety of more vigorous exercise for individuals with HCM, aged 8 to 60 years, with or without ICDs, as well as the impact of exercise on quality of life (available at: http://livehcm.org/).

Exercise and progression of disease in hypertrophic cardiomyopathy

Poor exercise capacity, measured by peak oxygen consumption, is associated with adverse outcomes in HCM, specifically the development of heart failure.[72] One study showed that LV outflow tract obstruction was associated with failure to augment stroke volume index and peak oxygen consumption.[73] In this study, the primary determinant of poor cardiac reserve was failure of stroke volume augmentation. In an earlier study, exercise-induced myocardial dysfunction was associated with clinical deterioration and worse outcomes.[74]

Although these studies show that poor exercise capacity is a predictor of adverse outcomes in HCM patients, whether exercise could accelerate or, on the other hand, attenuate the progression of disease, is unknown. An animal study by Konhilas and colleagues[75] showed that exercise prevented fibrosis, myocyte disarray, and induction of hypertrophic markers when initiated before established HCM disease. Also, when initiated in older animals with established HCM disease, exercise reversed myocyte disarray (but not fibrosis) and hypertrophic marker induction. Understanding the impact of exercise on the progression of HCM is an important avenue for further research.

Increasing exercise in the sedentary hypertrophic cardiomyopathy patient: Is it possible? Does it improve outcomes?

Although understanding safe levels of athletic participation and vigorous exercise is important, increasing the activity for sedentary HCM patients may be a more pressing issue for a large proportion of HMC patients. A survey by Reineck, Day and colleagues,[76] which compared HCM patients with participants in the National Health and Nutrition Examination Survey, found that patients with HCM reported less time engaged in physical activity at work and for leisure, and had a higher body mass index. An Australian study similarly reported that most HCM patients did not meet physical activity recommendations, and many participants reported that they had been advised not to exercise at all.[77]

Several studies have investigated the safety of exercise programs to increase fitness for patients with HCM, finding improved exercise capacity and no increase in arrhythmias. In a small pilot study, Klempfner and colleagues[78] evaluated the benefits and feasibility of increasing exercise in 20 symptomatic subjects with HCM who had significant limitation in their everyday activity. Subjects exercised in a cardiac rehabilitation center twice a week, using a treadmill, arm ergometer, and upright cycle exerciser. Their exercise prescription was based on heart rate reserve determined from a symptom-limited graded exercise stress test, during which a gradual increase in exercise intensity from 50% to 85% of the heart rate reserve over the training period was achieved. A significant improvement in functional capacity was noted (as assessed by a graded exercise test), and NYHA functional class improved from baseline by greater than or equal to 1 grade in 10 subjects (50%). During the study period and a follow-up of 12 months, none of the subjects experienced clinical deterioration or significant adverse events. This study suggests that moderate exercise may be not just safe but also beneficial in decreasing symptom burden. There are many possible pathways that may underlie the improvement in symptoms shown in these studies, which is that exercise improves diastolic function[79] and improves endothelial function.[80]

The large-scale randomized exploratory Study of exercise training in hypertrophic cardiomyopathy (RESET-HCM) study was the first randomized clinical trial of exercise for patients with HCM. In this study, moderate-intensity, unsupervised aerobic training versus usual activity was evaluated in 136 adults with HCM over a 4-month follow-up period. There was a statistically significant increase in the primary endpoint of change in mean peak oxygen consumption per unit time of greater than

1.35 mL/kg/min among the 67 subjects in the exercise group compared with greater than 0.08 mL/kg/min in the 66 subjects in the usual-activity group (**Fig. 6**). In the exploratory secondary endpoints, the premature ventricular contraction burden was reduced, with notable improvement in the physical functioning component of the quality-of-life scores in the exercise group. It was clear that the moderate exercise regimen used in this trial increased exercise capacity at 16 weeks without a signal for harm in terms of arrhythmic events or adverse remodeling.[81]

Dilated Cardiomyopathy

Clinical, pathologic, and genetic features of dilated cardiomyopathy (DCM) are beyond the scope of this article. In general, sudden death occurs in up to 12% of patients with this disorder and accounts for 25% to 30% of all deaths.[82,83] To what extent exercise may contribute to arrhythmias or progression of disease for patients with DCM has not been addressed. Moderate exercise, however, is recommended for those with heart failure in general. The 2013 AHA guidelines for management of heart failure[84] recommend exercise training (or regular physical activity) as safe and effective for patients with heart failure who are able to participate, to improve functional status (class I, level of evidence: A). The guidelines also state that cardiac rehabilitation is useful in clinically stable patients with heart failure to improve functional capacity, exercise duration, health-related quality of life, and mortality (class IIa, level of evidence: B). Although not specifically geared toward genetic DCM, those recommendations are obviously also relevant to this group.

No studies have investigated the effect of exercise in subjects with genetic DCM. However, because approximately 40% to 50% of DCM patients have an identifiable genetic cause, studies of structured exercise have been inclusive of this group. For example, in the study by Dougherty and colleagues[85] showing that prescription of home exercise is safe and effective in improving outcomes and cardiovascular performance in patients with DCM,[85] 48 subjects (30% of the study population) had nonischemic DCM. The large-scale A Controlled Trial Investigating Outcomes of Exercise Training (HF-ACTION) study, in which a modest but sustained improvement in quality of life with exercise was observed, included about half nonischemic cardiomyopathy.[86]

The safety versus risk of more vigorous exercise, such as athletic training or competition, for those with genetic DCM is not known.[65] The current recommendation is that symptomatic athletes with DCM should not participate in most competitive sports, with the possible exception of low-intensity (class 1A sports), at least until more information is available (class III; level of evidence C). It is not clear yet whether asymptomatic patients with DCM are at risk for sudden death during competitive athletics, because ventricular tachyarrhythmias are most common in patients with more advanced disease.[65] There are no current data regarding exercise in patients with positive genotype and negative phenotype.[65]

SUMMARY

Exercise has multiple benefits, both physical and psychological. Patients with these genetic cardiomyopathies can safely participate in low-intensity sports as recommended by AHA. With a multidisciplinary approach, shared decision-making, and taking the patient's priorities and preferences into account, a patient can gain many health benefits from exercise as opposed to a sedentary lifestyle. Patients with ARVC seem to be at higher risk of SCD and progression of disease with vigorous exercise, whereas HCM patients seem to benefit from at least a moderate intensity exercise regimen. Further data are needed on the safety of vigorous exercise for patients with HCM and DCM.

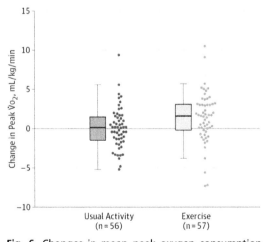

Fig. 6. Changes in mean peak oxygen consumption for HCM patients with usual activity versus exercise in the RESET-HCM study. (*From* Saberi S, Wheeler M, Bragg-Gresham J, et al. Effect of moderate-intensity exercise training on peak oxygen consumption in patients with hypertrophic cardiomyopathy: a randomized clinical trial. JAMA 2017;317(13):1349–57; with permission.)

REFERENCES

1. Statistics BoL. Percent of people aged 15 years and older who engaged in sports or exercise activities on

an average day, by region, 2003-06. Available at: https://www.bls.gov/spotlight/2008/sports/data.htm#chart01. Accessed October 27, 2017.

2. Bagnall RD, Weintraub RG, Ingles J, et al. A prospective study of sudden cardiac death among children and young adults. N Engl J Med 2016;374(25):2441–52.

3. Margey R, Roy A, Tobin S, et al. Sudden cardiac death in 14- to 35-year olds in Ireland from 2005 to 2007: a retrospective registry. Europace 2011; 13(10):1411–8.

4. Winkel BG, Holst AG, Theilade J, et al. Nationwide study of sudden cardiac death in persons aged 1-35 years. Eur Heart J 2011;32(8):983–90.

5. Toresdahl BG, Rao AL, Harmon KG, et al. Incidence of sudden cardiac arrest in high school student athletes on school campus. Heart Rhythm 2014;11(7): 1190–4.

6. Maron BJ, Doerer JJ, Haas TS, et al. Sudden deaths in young competitive athletes: analysis of 1866 deaths in the United States, 1980-2006. Circulation 2009;119(8):1085–92.

7. Risgaard B, Winkel BG, Jabbari R, et al. Sports-related sudden cardiac death in a competitive and a noncompetitive athlete population aged 12 to 49 years: data from an unselected nationwide study in Denmark. Heart Rhythm 2014;11(10):1673–81.

8. Landry CH, Allan KS, Connelly KA, et al. Sudden cardiac arrest during participation in competitive sports. N Engl J Med 2017;377(20):1943–53.

9. Harmon KG, Asif IM, Klossner D, et al. Incidence of sudden cardiac death in National Collegiate Athletic Association athletes. Circulation 2011;123(15): 1594–600.

10. Thiene G, Nava A, Corrado D, et al. Right ventricular cardiomyopathy and sudden death in young people. N Engl J Med 1988;318(3):129–33.

11. Finocchiaro G, Papadakis M, Robertus J-L, et al. Etiology of sudden death in sports: insights from a United Kingdom Regional Registry. J Am Coll Cardiol 2016;67(18):2108–15.

12. Harmon KG, Drezner JA, Maleszewski JJ, et al. Pathogeneses of sudden cardiac death in National Collegiate Athletic Association athletes. Circ Arrhythm Electrophysiol 2014;7(2):198–204.

13. Harmon KG, Asif IM, Maleszewski JJ, et al. Incidence, cause, and comparative frequency of sudden cardiac death in National Collegiate Athletic Association Athletes: a decade in review. Circulation 2015;132(1):10–9.

14. Marijon E, Uy-Evanado A, Reinier K, et al. Sudden cardiac arrest during sports activity in middle age. Circulation 2015;131(16):1384–91.

15. Lampert R, Olshansky B, Heidbuchel H, et al. Safety of sports for athletes with implantable cardioverter-defibrillators: results of a prospective, multinational registry. Circulation 2013;127(20):2021–30.

16. National Institutes of Health. Physical activity and cardiovascular health. NIH consensus development panel on physical activity and cardiovascular health. JAMA 1996;276(3):241–6.

17. Fletcher GF, Balady G, Blair SN, et al. Statement on exercise: benefits and recommendations for physical activity programs for all Americans. A statement for health professionals by the Committee on Exercise and Cardiac Rehabilitation of the Council on Clinical Cardiology, American Heart Association. Circulation 1996;94(4):857–62.

18. Physical Activity Guidelines Advisory Committee report, 2008. To the Secretary of Health and Human Services. Part A: executive summary. Nutr Rev 2009; 67(2):114–20.

19. Eckel RH, Jakicic JM, Ard JD, et al. 2013 AHA/ACC guideline on lifestyle management to reduce cardiovascular risk: a report of the American College of Cardiology/American Heart Association Task Force on Practice Guidelines. J Am Coll Cardiol 2014; 63(25 Pt B):2960–84.

20. Maessen MF, Verbeek AL, Bakker EA, et al. Lifelong exercise patterns and cardiovascular health. Mayo Clin Proc 2016;91(6):745–54.

21. Wen CP, Wai JP, Tsai MK, et al. Minimum amount of physical activity for reduced mortality and extended life expectancy: a prospective cohort study. Lancet 2011;378(9798):1244–53.

22. Macera CA, Hootman JM, Sniezek JE. Major public health benefits of physical activity. Arthritis Rheum 2003;49(1):122–8.

23. Macera CA, Powell KE. Population attributable risk: implications of physical activity dose. Med Sci Sports Exerc 2001;33(6 Suppl):S635–9 [discussion: 640–1].

24. Blair SN, Kohl HW 3rd, Paffenbarger RS Jr, et al. Physical fitness and all-cause mortality. A prospective study of healthy men and women. JAMA 1989; 262(17):2395–401.

25. Erikssen G, Liestol K, Bjornholt J, et al. Changes in physical fitness and changes in mortality. Lancet 1998;352(9130):759–62.

26. Yu S, Yarnell JW, Sweetnam PM, et al. What level of physical activity protects against premature cardiovascular death? The Caerphilly study. Heart 2003; 89(5):502–6.

27. Haskell WL, Lee IM, Pate RR, et al. Physical activity and public health: updated recommendation for adults from the American College of Sports Medicine and the American Heart Association. Circulation 2007;116(9):1081–93.

28. Paffenbarger RS Jr, Hyde RT, Wing AL, et al. Physical activity, all-cause mortality, and longevity of college alumni. N Engl J Med 1986;314(10):605–13.

29. Tanasescu M, Leitzmann MF, Rimm EB, et al. Exercise type and intensity in relation to coronary heart disease in men. JAMA 2002;288(16):1994–2000.

30. Sigal RJ, Kenny GP, Wasserman DH, et al. Physical activity/exercise and type 2 diabetes. Diabetes Care 2004;27(10):2518–39.

31. Kraus WE, Houmard JA, Duscha BD, et al. Effects of the amount and intensity of exercise on plasma lipoproteins. N Engl J Med 2002;347(19):1483–92.

32. Boule NG, Haddad E, Kenny GP, et al. Effects of exercise on glycemic control and body mass in type 2 diabetes mellitus: a meta-analysis of controlled clinical trials. JAMA 2001;286(10):1218–27.

33. Lachman S, Boekholdt SM, Luben RN, et al. Impact of physical activity on the risk of cardiovascular disease in middle-aged and older adults: EPIC Norfolk prospective population study. Eur J Prev Cardiol 2017;25(2):200–8.

34. Kriska A, Delahanty L, Edelstein S, et al. Sedentary behavior and physical activity in youth with recent onset of type 2 diabetes. Pediatrics 2013;131(3):e850–6.

35. Loprinzi PD, Lee IM, Andersen RE, et al. Association of concurrent healthy eating and regular physical activity with cardiovascular disease risk factors in U.S. youth. Am J Health Promot 2015;30(1):2–8.

36. Janssen I, Leblanc AG. Systematic review of the health benefits of physical activity and fitness in school-aged children and youth. Int J Behav Nutr Phys Act 2010;7:40.

37. Cuenca-Garcia M, Ortega FB, Ruiz JR, et al. Combined influence of healthy diet and active lifestyle on cardiovascular disease risk factors in adolescents. Scand J Med Sci Sports 2014; 24(3):553–62.

38. McAllister DR, Motamedi AR, Hame SL, et al. Quality of life assessment in elite collegiate athletes. Am J Sports Med 2001;29(6):806–10.

39. Snyder AR, Martinez JC, Bay RC, et al. Health-related quality of life differs between adolescent athletes and adolescent nonathletes. J Sport Rehabil 2010;19(3):237–48.

40. Malmberg J, Miilunpalo S, Pasanen M, et al. Characteristics of leisure time physical activity associated with risk of decline in perceived health–a 10-year follow-up of middle-aged and elderly men and women. Prev Med 2005;41(1):141–50.

41. Allgower A, Wardle J, Steptoe A. Depressive symptoms, social support, and personal health behaviors in young men and women. Health Psychol 2001; 20(3):223–7.

42. Anton SD, Newton RL Jr, Sothern M, et al. Association of depression with Body Mass Index, sedentary behavior, and maladaptive eating attitudes and behaviors in 11 to 13-year old children. Eat Weight Disord 2006;11(3):e102–8.

43. Brown RS. Exercise and mental health in the pediatric population. Clin Sports Med 1982;1(3):515–27.

44. Hoare E, Milton K, Foster C, et al. The associations between sedentary behaviour and mental health among adolescents: a systematic review. Int J Behav Nutr Phys Act 2016;13(1):108.

45. Rasberry CN, Lee SM, Robin L, et al. The association between school-based physical activity, including physical education, and academic performance: a systematic review of the literature. Prev Med 2011;52(Suppl 1):S10–20.

46. Michael SL, Merlo CL, Basch CE, et al. Critical connections: health and academics. J Sch Health 2015; 85(11):740–58.

47. Marzetti E, Calvani R, Tosato M, et al. Physical activity and exercise as countermeasures to physical frailty and sarcopenia. Aging Clin Exp Res 2017; 29(1):35–42.

48. Taylor D. Physical activity is medicine for older adults. Postgrad Med J 2014;90(1059):26–32.

49. Blondell SJ, Hammersley-Mather R, Veerman JL. Does physical activity prevent cognitive decline and dementia?: a systematic review and meta-analysis of longitudinal studies. BMC Public Health 2014;14:510.

50. Park SH, Han KS, Kang CB. Effects of exercise programs on depressive symptoms, quality of life, and self-esteem in older people: a systematic review of randomized controlled trials. Appl Nurs Res 2014; 27(4):219–26.

51. Lok N, Lok S, Canbaz M. The effect of physical activity on depressive symptoms and quality of life among elderly nursing home residents: Randomized controlled trial. Arch Gerontol Geriatr 2017;70: 92–8.

52. Perk J, De Backer G, Gohlke H, et al. European guidelines on cardiovascular disease prevention in clinical practice (version 2012). The fifth joint task force of the European Society of Cardiology and Other Societies on Cardiovascular Disease Prevention in Clinical Practice (constituted by representatives of nine societies and by invited experts). Eur Heart J 2012;33(13):1635–701.

53. Corrado D, Wichter T, Link MS, et al. Treatment of arrhythmogenic right ventricular cardiomyopathy/dysplasia: an international task force consensus statement. Circulation 2015;132(5):441–53.

54. Groeneweg JA, Bhonsale A, James CA, et al. Clinical presentation, long-term follow-up, and outcomes of 1001 arrhythmogenic right ventricular dysplasia/cardiomyopathy patients and family members. Circ Cardiovasc Genet 2015;8(3):437–46.

55. Protonotarios A, Anastasakis A, Panagiotakos DB, et al. Arrhythmic risk assessment in genotyped families with arrhythmogenic right ventricular cardiomyopathy. Europace 2016;18(4):610–6.

56. Zorzi A, Rigato I, Pilichou K, et al. Phenotypic expression is a prerequisite for malignant arrhythmic events and sudden cardiac death in arrhythmogenic right ventricular cardiomyopathy. Europace 2016; 18(7):1086–94.

57. Corrado D, Basso C, Thiene G, et al. Spectrum of clinicopathologic manifestations of arrhythmogenic right ventricular cardiomyopathy/dysplasia: a multicenter study. J Am Coll Cardiol 1997;30(6):1512–20.

58. Lampert R, Olshansky B, Heidbuchel H, et al. Safety of sports for athletes with implantable cardioverter-defibrillators: long-term results of a prospective multinational registry. Circulation 2017;135(23):2310–2.

59. James CA, Bhonsale A, Tichnell C, et al. Exercise increases age-related penetrance and arrhythmic risk in arrhythmogenic right ventricular dysplasia/cardiomyopathy-associated desmosomal mutation carriers. J Am Coll Cardiol 2013;62(14):1290–7.

60. Ruwald AC, Marcus F, Estes NA 3rd, et al. Association of competitive and recreational sport participation with cardiac events in patients with arrhythmogenic right ventricular cardiomyopathy: results from the North American multidisciplinary study of arrhythmogenic right ventricular cardiomyopathy. Eur Heart J 2015;36(27):1735–43.

61. Sawant AC, Te Riele AS, Tichnell C, et al. Safety of American Heart Association-recommended minimum exercise for desmosomal mutation carriers. Heart Rhythm 2016;13(1):199–207.

62. Mazzanti A, Ng K, Faragli A, et al. Arrhythmogenic right ventricular cardiomyopathy: clinical course and predictors of arrhythmic risk. J Am Coll Cardiol 2016;68(23):2540–50.

63. La Gerche A, Heidbuchel H, Burns AT, et al. Disproportionate exercise load and remodeling of the athlete's right ventricle. Med Sci Sports Exerc 2011;43(6):974–81.

64. Kirchhof P, Fabritz L, Zwiener M, et al. Age- and training-dependent development of arrhythmogenic right ventricular cardiomyopathy in heterozygous plakoglobin-deficient mice. Circulation 2006;114(17):1799–806.

65. Maron BJ, Udelson JE, Bonow RO, et al. Eligibility and disqualification recommendations for competitive athletes with cardiovascular abnormalities: task force 3: hypertrophic cardiomyopathy, arrhythmogenic right ventricular cardiomyopathy and other cardiomyopathies, and myocarditis: a scientific statement from the American Heart Association and American College of Cardiology. Circulation 2015;132(22):e273–80.

66. Sawant AC, Bhonsale A, te Riele AS, et al. Exercise has a disproportionate role in the pathogenesis of arrhythmogenic right ventricular dysplasia/cardiomyopathy in patients without desmosomal mutations. J Am Heart Assoc 2014;3(6):e001471.

67. Maron BJ, Rowin EJ, Casey SA, et al. Hypertrophic Cardiomyopathy in children, adolescents, and young adults associated with low cardiovascular mortality with contemporary management strategies. Circulation 2016;133(1):62–73.

68. Maron BJ, Rowin EJ, Casey SA, et al. Risk stratification and outcome of patients with hypertrophic cardiomyopathy >=60 years of age. Circulation 2013;127(5):585–93.

69. Gersh BJ, Maron BJ, Bonow RO, et al. 2011 ACCF/AHA guideline for the diagnosis and treatment of hypertrophic cardiomyopathy: a report of the American College of Cardiology Foundation/American Heart Association Task Force on Practice Guidelines. Circulation 2011;124(24):e783–831.

70. Authors/Task Force members, Elliott PM, Anastasakis A, Borger MA, et al. 2014 ESC Guidelines on diagnosis and management of hypertrophic cardiomyopathy: the Task Force for the Diagnosis and Management of Hypertrophic Cardiomyopathy of the European Society of Cardiology (ESC). Eur Heart J 2014;35(39):2733–79.

71. Pelliccia A, Corrado D, Bjornstad HH, et al. Recommendations for participation in competitive sport and leisure-time physical activity in individuals with cardiomyopathies, myocarditis and pericarditis. Eur J Cardiovasc Prev Rehabil 2006;13(6):876–85.

72. Coats CJ, Rantell K, Bartnik A, et al. Cardiopulmonary exercise testing and prognosis in hypertrophic cardiomyopathy. Circ Heart Fail 2015;8(6):1022–31.

73. Critoph CH, Patel V, Mist B, et al. Cardiac output response and peripheral oxygen extraction during exercise among symptomatic hypertrophic cardiomyopathy patients with and without left ventricular outflow tract obstruction. Heart 2014;100(8):639–46.

74. Pelliccia F, Cianfrocca C, Pristipino C, et al. Cumulative exercise-induced left ventricular systolic and diastolic dysfunction in hypertrophic cardiomyopathy. Int J Cardiol 2007;122(1):76–8.

75. Konhilas JP, Watson PA, Maass A, et al. Exercise can prevent and reverse the severity of hypertrophic cardiomyopathy. Circ Res 2006;98(4):540–8.

76. Reineck E, Rolston B, Bragg-Gresham JL, et al. Physical activity and other health behaviors in adults with hypertrophic cardiomyopathy. Am J Cardiol 2013;111:1034–9.

77. Sweeting J, Ingles J, Timperio I, et al. Physical inactivity in hypertrophic cardiomyopathy: prevalence of inactivity and perceived barriers. Open Heart 2016;3:e000484.

78. Klempfner R, Kamerman T, Schwammenthal E, et al. Efficacy of exercise training in symptomatic patients with hypertrophic cardiomyopathy: results of a structured exercise training program in a cardiac rehabilitation center. Eur J Prev Cardiol 2015;22(1):13–9.

79. Edelmann F, Gelbrich G, Düngen H-D, et al. Exercise training improves exercise capacity and diastolic function in patients with heart failure with preserved ejection fraction: results of the Ex-DHF (Exercise training in Diastolic Heart Failure) pilot study. J Am Coll Cardiol 2011;58(17):1780–91.

80. Gevaert AB, Lemmens K, Vrints CJ, et al. Targeting endothelial function to treat heart failure with preserved ejection fraction: the promise of exercise training. Oxid Med Cell Longev 2017;2017:4865756.

81. Saberi S, Wheeler M, Bragg-Gresham J, et al. Effect of moderate-intensity exercise training on peak oxygen consumption in patients with hypertrophic cardiomyopathy: a randomized clinical trial. JAMA 2017;317(13):1349–57.

82. Dec GW, Fuster V. Idiopathic dilated cardiomyopathy. N Engl J Med 1994;331(23):1564–75.

83. Broch K, Murbraech K, Andreassen AK, et al. Contemporary outcome in patients with idiopathic dilated cardiomyopathy. Am J Cardiol 2015;116(6):952–9.

84. Yancy CW, Jessup M, Bozkurt B, et al. 2013 ACCF/AHA guideline for the management of heart failure: a report of the American College of Cardiology Foundation/American Heart Association Task Force on Practice Guidelines. J Am Coll Cardiol 2013; 62(16):e147–239.

85. Dougherty CM, Glenny RW, Burr RL, et al. Prospective randomized trial of moderately strenuous aerobic exercise after an implantable cardioverter defibrillator. Circulation 2015;131(21):1835–42.

86. Flynn KE, Pina IL, Whellan DJ, et al. Effects of exercise training on health status in patients with chronic heart failure: HF-ACTION randomized controlled trial. JAMA 2009;301(14):1451–9.

Diagnostic Criteria, Genetics, and Molecular Basis of Arrhythmogenic Cardiomyopathy

Cristina Basso, MD, PhD*, Kalliopi Pilichou, PhD,
Barbara Bauce, MD, PhD, Domenico Corrado, MD, PhD,
Gaetano Thiene, MD

KEYWORDS

- Arrhythmogenic right ventricular cardiomyopathy • Desmosomes • Sudden cardiac death
- Implantable cardioverter defibrillator

KEY POINTS

- Clinical presentation is characterized by ventricular arrhythmias at risk of sudden death. More rarely, right ventricular or biventricular dysfunction leading to heart failure is reported
- Generally referred as right ventricular disease, recognition of left-dominant and biventricular subtypes prompted the use of the broader term AC.
- Effort is a trigger of disease onset and progression as well as ventricular arrhythmias.
- Disease causing genes mostly encode for desmosomal proteins, although non-desmosomal genes are also described.
- Knowledge of phenocopies that can mimic AC is essential to avoid misdiagnosis.

Arrhythmogenic cardiomyopathy (AC) is an inherited, genetically determined heart muscle disease characterized by myocardial atrophy with fibrofatty repair. It usually manifests with electrocardiographic (ECG) abnormalities, syncope, or ventricular arrhythmias during adolescence or young adulthood.[1–5] AC represents one of the major causes of sudden death in the young and athletes.[1,6] The disease is listed among rare cardiovascular disorders, because its estimated prevalence in the general population ranges from 1:2000 to 1:5000.[7,8]

The structural substrate of AC consists of myocardial atrophy, which occurs progressively with time, through periodic "acute bursts" of an otherwise stable disease, starting from the epicardium and eventually extending down to reach the endocardium to become transmural ("wave-front phenomenon"). Myocyte necrosis is seldom evident, as a proof of the acquired and progressive nature of myocardial atrophy. Myocardial inflammation has been reported in up to 75% of autoptic AC hearts and probably plays a role in triggering life-threatening ventricular tachyarrhythmias.

Right ventricular (RV) aneurysms, whether single or multiple, located in the so-called triangle of dysplasia (ie, inflow, apex, and outflow tract), are pathognomonic features of AC, although not always present.[1,2] Nevertheless, apparently normal hearts have been reported in which only a careful histopathology investigation can reveal fibrofatty

Disclosure Statement: The authors have nothing to disclose.
Department of Cardiac, Thoracic, and Vascular Sciences, University of Padova Medical School, Padova, Italy
* Corresponding author. Department of Cardiac Thoracic and Vascular Sciences, University of Padua Medical School, Via Gabelli, Padova 61-35121, Italy.
E-mail address: cristina.basso@unipd.it

Heart Failure Clin 14 (2018) 201–213
https://doi.org/10.1016/j.hfc.2018.01.002
1551-7136/18/© 2018 Elsevier Inc. All rights reserved.

replacement, in the absence of wall thinning, aneurysm, and chamber dilatation. Cases with isolated or predominant left ventricular (LV) involvement are increasingly detected.

Genetic studies have led to the identification of more than 10 disease-causative genes associated with AC. Nearly half of AC patients harbor mutations in genes encoding desmosomal proteins and less than 1% in non–desmosomal genes.[7]

With the gradual understanding of the genetic basis of the disease, the original name "dysplasia" was no longer considered proper and the term "cardiomyopathy" was introduced.[1–5,8] Moreover, because similar pathologic changes and arrhythmic manifestations may also occur in the setting of predominant involvement of the left ventricle,[9] the preferred disease name is now simply AC.

CLINICAL FEATURES

Clinical manifestations vary with age and disease stage. Despite the similar prevalence of mutation carriers in both genders, the clinical expression of the disease is usually more severe in men, with a higher prevalence of male than female patients who fulfill the diagnostic criteria (up to 3:1).[3,5] Palpitations, syncope, and cardiac arrest are common symptoms in young adults or adolescents, and the most typical signs of AC are ventricular arrhythmias with left bundle branch block (LBBB) morphology (either premature ventricular complexes or ventricular tachycardia [VT]) and T-wave inversion in precordial leads in the 12-lead ECG. Less common are RV and biventricular dilatation, with or without heart failure, mimicking dilated cardiomyopathy and requiring heart transplantation at the end stage.

Not infrequently, the patient can present with a myocarditis or a myocardial infarction-like picture with chest pain, dynamic ST-T wave changes on the 12-lead ECG, and myocardial enzyme release in the setting of normal coronary arteries.[3]

Traditionally, 4 clinical phases have been described in the classic RV variant of AC and include the following: (a) a concealed phase, with subtle RV structural changes, with or without ventricular arrhythmias, during which sudden death may even be the first manifestation of the disease; (b) an overt electrical phase, with symptomatic life-threatening ventricular arrhythmias associated with clear-cut RV morphofunctional abnormalities; (c) RV failure, due to progression and extension of the RV disease; and (d) biventricular failure, caused by advanced LV disease.[10] Sudden death due to electrical instability can occur at any time during the course of the disease.[3,5,6,11,12] The

incidence of sudden death ranges from 0.08% to 3.6% per year in adults with AC.[3,5,11]

Although scar-related reentry VT is the most frequent event in patients with an overt phenotype, ventricular fibrillation (VF) can occur in patients with an early stage or "hot phase" of the disease because of acute myocyte death and inflammation.[11,12] A possible role of gap junction remodeling with sodium channel interference has been also advanced to account for life-threatening arrhythmias.[13,14]

DIAGNOSTIC CRITERIA

Because there is no single gold standard, AC diagnosis requires multiple criteria, combining different sources of diagnostic information, such as morphofunctional (by echocardiography and/or angiography and/or cardiac magnetic resonance [CMR]), histopathological on endomyocardial biopsy, ECG, arrhythmias, and familial history, including genetics (**Fig. 1**).

The original diagnostic criteria[15] were revised in 2010[16] to improve diagnostic sensitivity, by maintaining diagnostic specificity (**Box 1**). Quantitative parameters have been included and abnormalities defined, based on the comparison with normal subject data. Moreover, T-wave inversion in V_1-V_3, and VT with a LBBB morphology with superior or indeterminate QRS axis (either sustained or no sustained), have become major diagnostic criteria[17]; T-wave inversion in V_1-V_2 in the absence of right bundle branch block (RBBB), and in V_1-V_4, in the presence of complete RBBB, has been included among the minor criteria (**Fig. 2**). Finally, major criteria in the family history category include the confirmation of AC in a first-degree relative, either by fulfilling the criteria or pathologically (at autopsy or transplantation), and the identification of a pathogenic mutation, categorized as associated or probably associated with AC. However, caution is recommended because the pathogenic significance of a single mutation is increasingly questioned, particularly in the era of next generation sequencing (NGS).

The diagnostic criteria are also valid in the pediatric age group, with the only exception of inverted T wave in right precordial leads in children less than 12 years of age, which is often normal. Noteworthy, AC diagnosis is exceptionally made younger than the age of 10 because of the age-related penetrance of the disease.[3,5]

After 2010, the exploding use of contrast-enhanced CMR in the routine clinical workup increasingly revealed left dominant variants of AC that escape clinical identification through current diagnostic criteria, thus underlying their limitations

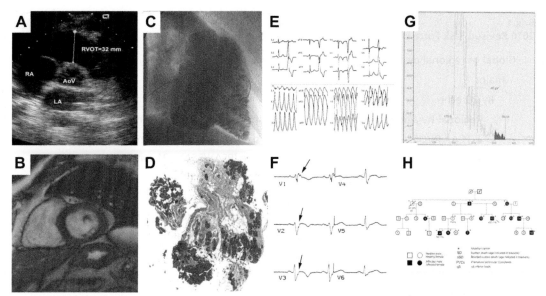

Fig. 1. The diagnosis of AC as a multiparametric approach in the classical RV variant: (*A, B, C*) echocardiography, CMR, and angiography showing RV dilatation and aneurysms; (*D*) tissue characterization through endomyocardial biopsy (H&E, original magnification ×5); (*E*) 12-lead ECG with inverted T waves V1-V3, LBBB morphology premature ventricular complexes and VT; (*F*) postexcitation epsilon wave in precordial leads V1-V3 (*arrows*); (*G*) signal-averaged ECG with late potentials (40-Hz high-pass filtering); (*H*) family pedigree with autosomal-dominant inheritance of the disease. AoV, aortic valve; LA, left atrium; RA, right atrium.

to this perspective (see **Fig. 2**; **Fig. 3**). In fact, the revised 2010 criteria can easily recognize RV and biventricular AC but lack specific diagnostic guidelines for the nonclassical LV disease pattern. ECG abnormalities, such as lateral or inferolateral T-wave inversion (leads V_5, V_6, L_I, and aVL), low-voltage QRS complex on peripheral leads, and RBBB/polymorphic ventricular arrhythmias suggest a left-sided involvement.[18] Moreover, noninvasive tissue characterization through late gadolinium enhancement, which is not included among the criteria, is by far a more-sensitive indicator of even early or minor left-sided disease. It typically involves the inferolateral and inferoseptal regions and affects the subepicardial or midwall layers (so-called nonischemic LV scars).[9,19,20] The absence of transmurality explains why it is detected frequently in a segment without a concomitant morphofunctional wall-motion abnormality, thus preceding the onset of LV dysfunction or dilatation, which is usually identified by traditional cardiac imaging.

Differential diagnosis with dilated cardiomyopathy and chronic myocarditis is mandatory for risk stratification and family screening.[21,22] Although LV AC has a propensity to electrical instability that exceeds the degree of ventricular dysfunction, dilated cardiomyopathy usually presents with life-threatening ventricular arrhythmias in the setting of low ejection fraction (<35%). Moreover,

a regional rather than global involvement is more in keeping with AC, particularly when RV abnormalities are prominent.

Differential Diagnosis

Myocarditis, sarcoidosis, RV infarction, dilated cardiomyopathy, Chagas disease, Brugada syndrome, idiopathic RV outflow tract VT, pulmonary hypertension, and congenital heart diseases with right chambers overload are the so-called clinical phenocopies, because they can mimic AC due to overlapping clinical symptoms and signs.[3] As a general principle, even more attention should be paid in not using a single parameter but to complement imaging, ECG, and family history information.

In selected cases, endomyocardial biopsy from the RV free wall can be crucial to reach the final diagnosis, ruling out myocarditis and sarcoidosis, especially when dealing with probands with sporadic forms, and in the setting of negative or doubtful CMR and/or electrovoltage mapping.[23,24] Replacement-type fibrosis, including some inflammatory infiltrates, myocyte degeneration, and evidence of adipogenesis, is a microscopic hallmark of AC.[23] Based on the current endomyocardial biopsy guidelines, fibrous or fibrofatty replacement with less than 60% residual myocardium in at least one endomyocardial biopsy sample is a major criterion, and 60% to 75% residual myocardium is a

Box 1
2010 Revised Task Force criteria for arrhythmogenic cardiomyopathy

I. Global or regional dysfunction and structural alterations[a]

   Major

   By 2D echo

   Regional RV akinesia, dyskinesia, or aneurysm and 1 of the following (end-diastole):

   - PLAX RVOT $\geq$32 mm [corrected for body size (PLAX/BSA) $\geq$19 mm/m^2]
   - PSAX RVOT $\geq$36 mm [corrected for body size (PSAX/BSA) $\geq$21 mm/m^2]
   - Or fractional area change $\leq$33%

   By CMR

   Regional RV akinesia or dyskinesia or dyssynchronous RV contraction and 1 of the following:

   - Ratio of RV end-diastolic volume to BSA $\geq$110 mL/m^2 (male) or $\geq$100 mL/m^2 (female)
   - Or RV ejection fraction $\leq$40%

   By RV angiography

   Regional RV akinesia, dyskinesia, or aneurysm

   Minor

   By 2D echo

   Regional RV akinesia or dyskinesia and 1 of the following (end diastole):

   - PLAX RVOT $\geq$29 to less than 32 mm [corrected for body size (PLAX/BSA) $\geq$16 to <19 m/m^2]
   - PSAX RVOT $\geq$32 to less than 36 mm [corrected for body size (PSAX/BSA) $\geq$18 to <21 mm/m^2]
   - Or fractional area change greater than 33% to $\leq$40%

   By CMR

   Regional RV akinesia or dyskinesia or dyssynchronous RV contraction and 1 of the following:

   - Ratio of RV end-diastolic volume to BSA $\geq$100 to less than 110 mL/m^2 (male) or $\geq$90 to less than 100 mL/m^2 (female)
   - Or RV ejection fraction greater than 40% to $\leq$45%

II. Tissue characterization of wall

   Major

   Fibrofatty replacement of myocardium on endomyocardial biopsy

   Residual myocytes <60% by morphometric analysis (or <50% if estimated), with fibrous replacement of the RV free wall myocardium in $\geq$1 sample, with or without fatty replacement of tissue on EMB

   Minor

   Residual myocytes <60% by morphometric analysis (or <50% if estimated), with fibrous replacement of the RV free wall myocardium in $\geq$1 sample, with or without fatty replacement of tissue on EMB

III. Repolarization abnormalities

   Major

   - Inverted T waves in right precordial leads (V1, V2, and V3) or beyond in individuals older than 14 years of age (in the absence of complete RBBB QRS $\geq$120 ms)

   Minor

   - Inverted T waves in leads V1 and V2 in individuals older than 14 years of age (in the absence of complete RBBB) or in V4, V5, or V6
   - Inverted T waves in leads V1, V2, V3, and V4 in individuals older than 14 years of age in the presence of complete RBBB

IV. Depolarization/conduction abnormalities

Major

- Epsilon wave (reproducible low-amplitude signals between end of QRS complex to onset of the T wave) in the right precordial leads (V1 to V3)

Minor

- Late potentials by SAECG in ≥1 of 3 parameters in the absence of a QRS duration of ≥110 ms on the standard ECG
- Filtered QRS duration ≥114 ms
- Duration of terminal QRS less than 40 µV (low-amplitude signal duration) ≥38 ms
- Root-mean-square voltage of terminal 40 ms ≤20 µV
- Terminal activation duration of QRS ≥55 ms measured from the nadir of the S wave to the end of the QRS, including R', in V1, V2, or V3, in the absence of complete RBBB

V. Arrhythmias

Major

- Nonsustained or sustained VT of LBBB morphology with superior axis (negative or indeterminate QRS in leads II, III, and aVF and positive in lead aVL)

Minor

- Nonsustained or sustained VT of RVOT, LBBB morphology with inferior axis (positive QRS in leads II, III, and aVF and negative in lead aVL), or of unknown axis
- >500 PVCs per 24 hours (Holter)

VI. Family history

Major

- AC confirmed in a first-degree relative who meets current Task Force criteria
- AC confirmed pathologically at autopsy or surgery in a first-degree relative
- Identification of a pathogenic mutation categorized as associated or probably associated with AC in the patient under evaluation

Minor

- History of AC in a first-degree relative in whom it is not possible or practical to determine whether the family member meets current Task Force criteria

  ○ Premature sudden death (35 years of age) due to suspected AC in a first-degree relative

  ○ AC confirmed pathologically or by current Task Force criteria in second-degree relative

Two major, or 1 major and 2 minor, or 4 minor criteria from different categories: definite AC diagnosis. One major and 1 minor, or 3 minor criteria: borderline AC diagnosis. One major of 2 minor criteria: possible AC diagnosis.
A pathogenic mutation is a DNA alteration associated with AC that alters or is expected to alter the encoded protein, is unobserved or rare in a large non-AC control population, and either alters or is predicted to alter the structure or function of the protein or has demonstrated linkage to the disease phenotype in a conclusive pedigree.
Abbreviations: BSA, body surface area; CMR, cardiac magnetic resonance; EMB, endomyocardial biopsy; LBBB, left bundle- branch block; PLAX, parasternal long-axis view; PSAX, parasternal short-axis view; PVC, premature ventricular complex; RBBB, right bundle-branch block; RV, right ventricle; RVOT, RV outflow tract; SD, sudden death; SAECG, Signal Average ECG; VT, ventricular tachycardia.
[a] Hypokinesis is not included in the definition of RV regional wall motion abnormalities in the proposed modified criteria.

minor criterion for AC. Electrovoltage mapping is an invasive electrophysiological tool that should be performed in selected patients with suspected AC, in the setting of ventricular arrhythmias of RV origin, and/or when contrast-enhanced CMR is negative or doubtful in terms of RV involvement.[24,25]

Another diagnostic pitfall is represented by idiopathic RV outflow tract VT, which is typically benign. The idiopathic nature of the VT is supported by some "red flags," such as the absence of ECG repolarization/depolarization abnormalities and of ventricular structural changes, the recording of a single VT morphology, noninducibility at

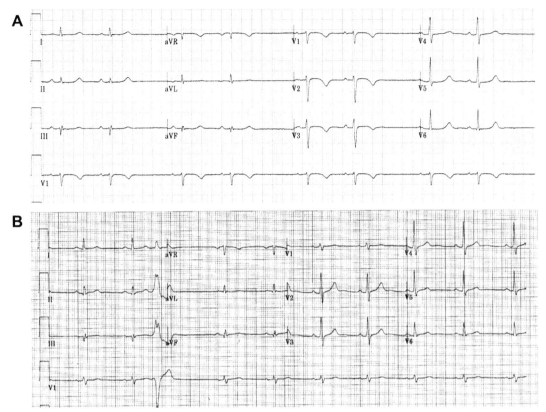

Fig. 2. ECG features of classical RV AC and LV AC variant. (*A*) Negative T waves in V1-V3 and low QRS voltage; (*B*) normal 12-lead ECG tracing in a DSP mutation carrier.

programmed ventricular stimulation, together with the nonfamilial background.[24] The identification of a structural substrate in the RV outflow tract is crucial to the diagnosis of AC, because abnormal low-voltage areas correspond to the loss of electrically active myocardium caused by fibrofatty replacement. However, in early stages of the disease, scar tissue may be confined to epicardial/midmural layers, sparing (or reaching focally) the endocardial region. Thus, bipolar endocardial voltage mapping of the RV free wall may underestimate or miss non-transmural low-voltage areas.[26]

Finally, a special consideration deserves the differential diagnosis between AC and athlete's heart in people performing sport activity. Physiologic adaptation to training with hemodynamic overload during exercise may account for RV enlargement, ECG abnormalities, and arrhythmias in endurance athletes.[3] Global RV systolic dysfunction and/or regional wall motion abnormalities, such as bulgings or aneurysms, are more in keeping with AC.[27,28] On the other hand, the absence of overt structural changes of the RV, frequent premature ventricular complexes (PVCs), or inverted T waves in the precordial leads all support a benign nature.

GENETICS

Although AC has been recognized as an inherited disease since the 1980s,[29] the first disease-causing gene was identified in 2000, when the investigations carried out on a similar disorder in the Naxos Island marked the turning point in the understanding of the genetic background. In a cohort of people with palmoplantar keratoderma, wooly hair, and AC cosegregating in a recessive pattern, a haplotype on chromosome 17q21 was first identified, and further analysis led to the discovery of a homozygous frameshift mutation (c.2040_2041delGT) in *JUP*, encoding plakoglobin.[30,31]

At the same time, mutations of the DSP gene were found to cause another autosomal-recessive cardiocutaneous syndrome, that is, Carvajal syndrome.[32] Only 2 years later, heterozygous mutations in the same gene were identified in an Italian family affected with a dominant form of AC without hair/skin abnormalities.[33] To date, different disease genes have been linked to the classical inheritance pattern of AC, highlighting genetic heterogeneity.[7] Most of the mutations in

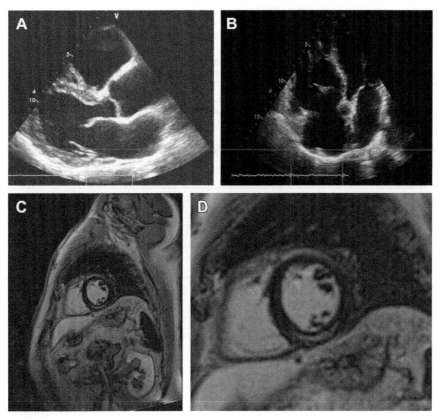

Fig. 3. Imaging features of classical RV AC and LV AC variant. (*A, B*) Severe RV dilatation and abnormal LV dimension and function (2D echo, parasternal long-axis view, and apical 4-chamber view) (same case as **Fig. 2**A). (*C, D*) Contrast-enhanced CMR: a subepicardial stria of gadolinium enhancement in the LV posterolateral wall in the setting of normal ventricular size and function (same case as **Fig. 2**B).

the dominant forms have been identified in desmosomal genes, including DSP, plakophilin-2 (PKP2), desmoglein-2 (DSG2), desmocollin-2 (DSC2), and JUP[33–37] (**Table 1**). Only isolated reports are on nondesmosome genes, such as transmembrane protein 43 (TMEM43), desmin (DES), titin (TTN), lamin A/C (LMNA), phospholamban (PLN), αT-catenin, filamin C (FLNC), N-cadherin (CDH2). Because their clinical picture is not always that of classical AC, they are often called phenocopies or overlap syndromes.[38–45] Moreover, mutations in the regulatory region of the transforming growth factor β-3 gene have been reported.[46]

Overall, pathogenic mutations mostly involve structural proteins of the intercalated disc, described as containing a mixed-type junctional structure instead of classical adherens junctions, the so-called area composita.[47]

Comprehensive exomic sequence analysis currently identifies desmosomal gene mutations in approximately 50% of AC probands.[7,48–53] PKP2 is the most commonly defective AC gene (10%–45%), followed by DSP (10%–15%), DSG2 (7%–10%), and DSC2, JUP (1%–2%). Compound, heterozygous mutations are present in 10% to 25% of AC patients.[7,49–51] Although "private" mutations predominate in AC patients, founder mutations in both desmosomal and extra-desmosomal encoding genes have been reported.[7,52] We recently identified genomic rearrangements in ≈7% of AC probands negative for pathogenic point mutations in desmosomal genes,[53] thus highlighting the potential of copy number variations analysis to substantially increase the diagnostic yield of genetic testing and expanding previous observations.[54] Several factors can account for the variability in genotyping success rate, such as cohort location and ethnicity, sequencing techniques, selection, and stringency of criteria to define causative mutations. Moreover, the routine use of NGS for the analysis of large panels of genes or even the analysis of the whole exome is leading to the identification of a large number of nucleotide variants with uncertain clinical significance. Genetic testing and its interpretation should be performed by geneticists in

Table 1
Genetic background of arrhythmogenic cardiomyopathy

MIM Entry	Locus	Disease Gene	Gene	Mode of Transmission	Author, Year	Comment
Desmosomal genes						
#611528 #601214	17q21.2	Plakoglobin	JUP	AD/AR	McKoy et al,[31] 2000	AR form: cardiocutaneous syndrome
#607450 #605676	6p24.3	Desmoplakin	DSP	AD/AR	Rampazzo et al,[33] 2002	AR form: cardiocutaneous syndrome
#609040	12p11.21	Plakophilin-2	PKP2	AD/AR	Gerull et al,[34] 2005	
#610193	18q12.1	Desmoglein-2	DSG2	AD/AR	Pilichou et al,[35] 2006	
#610476	18q12.1	Desmocollin-2	DSC2	AD/AR	Syrris et al,[36] 2006	
Nondesmosomal genes						
#107970	14q24.3	Transforming growth factor-β-3	TGFB3	AD	Beffagna et al,[46] 2005	Modifier?
#604400	3p25.1	Transmembrane protein 43	TMEM43	AD	Merner et al,[38] 2008	
	2q35	Desmin	DES	AD	van Tintelen et al,[39] 2009	Overlap syndrome (DC and HC phenotype, early conduction disease)
	6q22.31	Phospholamban	PLN	AD	van der Zwaag et al,[40] 2010	
	2q31.2	Titin	TTN	AD	Taylor et al,[41] 2011	Overlap syndrome (early conduction disease, AF)
	1q22	Lamin A/C	LMNA	AD	Quarta et al,[42] 2012	Overlap syndrome
#615616	10q21.3	α-T-catenin	CTNAA3	AD	van Hengel et al,[43] 2013	
	7q32.1	Filamin C	FLNC	AD	Ortiz-Genga et al,[44] 2016	Overlap syndrome (HC and DC phenotype)
	18q12.1	N-Cadherin	CDH2	AD	Mayosi et al,[45] 2017	

Abbreviations: AD, autosomal dominant; AF, atrial fibrillation; AR, autosomal recessive; DC, dilated cardiomyopathy; HC, hypertrophic cardiomyopathy; MIM, Mendelian Inheritance in Man.

dedicated AC cardiogenetic centers, with precounseling and postcounseling facilities.[51]

Early genotype-phenotype correlation studies, mostly based on a few families, separately addressed mutations in different desmosomal genes and compared clinical manifestations of AC mutation carriers versus noncarriers.[55,56] Although some differences have been reported with regard to a series of clinical, ECG, and morphofunctional RV abnormalities, detection of AC desmosomal gene mutations was not associated with a higher susceptibility to life-threatening arrhythmias and did not predict arrhythmic outcome.

Few available publications correlating the phenotype to the genotype provided contradictory findings with regard to the association between specific desmosomal genes or mutations and clinical features. DSP was originally reported as a gene of arrhythmogenic LV cardiomyopathy or dominant AC,[18,57] and a specific trend toward more prevalent LV involvement was attributed to *DSP* mutations by Quarta and colleagues[58] and to *DSG-2* mutations by Fressart and colleagues.[59]

In our series of 134 desmosomal gene mutation carriers, disease penetrance did not differ according to specific desmosomal genes or to the presence of missense versus non-missense mutations.[49] Carriers of single non-missense mutations significantly more often had right precordial T-wave inversion extending beyond lead V3 and showed a trend toward a lower mean RV fractional area change compared with carriers of single missense mutations. No statistically significant differences in the clinical phenotype were attributable to specific desmosomal genes, with the exception of *DSP* gene mutation carriers who distinctively had more frequent negative T waves confined to leads V4 to V6, low QRS voltages in limb leads, and LV dysfunction with ejection fraction. Finally, disease penetrance was higher in patients with multiple mutations than in those with single mutations.

Similar data were reported in the large US and Dutch AC cohorts, with pathogenic mutations in desmosomal and nondesmosomal genes identified in 577 patients.[52] In fact, individuals with more than one mutation have considerably worse clinical course with significantly earlier onset of symptoms and first sustained arrhythmia, a greater chance of developing sustained VT/VF, and a 5-fold increase in the risk of developing LV dysfunction and heart failure than those carrying a single mutation. Among carriers of a single mutation, this study demonstrated that the risk of LV involvement and development of heart failure is intrinsically related to the mutated gene. Conversely, carriers of single mutations in all the genes had a high risk of developing a life-threatening arrhythmia, with no significant differences in VT/VF survival among the different genes. PLN mutation carriers had an older age of presentation, although they showed a worse long-term prognosis, with more LV dysfunction and heart failure. Also, DSP mutation carriers were more likely to develop heart failure and signs of LV involvement, confirming the observation from prior smaller cohorts. These investigators also provided evidence that missense variants, defined as pathogenic by predicting algorithms, are associated with a similar prognosis as premature truncating or splice site mutations.

On the basis of these preliminary data, compound or digenic (compound/digenic heterozygosity) desmosomal mutations, which account for up to 25% of AC patient in different series, are now considered in the risk stratification for the prevention of sudden cardiac death.[12]

PATHOGENESIS

Experimental animal and cellular models are useful tools to explore how mutant desmosomal proteins lead to cardiomyocyte death and subsequent repair with fibrous and fatty tissue.[4,7,60,61]

Abnormal Cell-Cell Adhesion

Ultrastructural studies demonstrating intercalated disc remodeling first raised the hypothesis of an abnormal cellular adhesion in disease pathogenesis.[62] Abnormal cell-cell adhesion would predispose myocytes to detachment, death, and replacement by fibrofatty tissue. Exercise exacerbates this adhesion defect, particularly at the level of the thinner RV wall as compared with the LV wall. The role of exercise as a disease modifier has been demonstrated in multiple murine models and was confirmed by clinical studies of desmosomal-gene mutations carriers.[63] Noteworthy, mutation carriers engaged in endurance sports are symptomatic earlier, have a higher tendency to develop an overt phenotype, and show a worse prognosis.

Abnormal Signaling Pathways

Desmosomes are important mediators of intracellular and intercellular signal transduction pathways, besides being specialized structures for mechanical cell-to-cell attachment. The role of canonical Wnt/β-catenin/Tcf/Lef signaling pathway suppression, as a consequence of the abnormal distribution of intercalated disc proteins, was first demonstrated by Garcia-Gras and colleagues[64] in a Dsp-deficient mouse model. It is a well-known regulator of adipogenesis, fibrogenesis, and apoptosis. Knockdown of DSP in HL-1 cells causes the translocation of JUP into the nucleus, where it interferes with β-catenin/TCF transcriptional activity, leading to an adipogenic switch.

Further confirming the role of canonical Wnt in AC pathogenesis is the efficacy of therapies designed to increase Wnt signaling. A chemical screen with zebrafish expressing plakoglobin mutation identified SB216763, an inhibitor of glycogen synthase kinase 3-β (GSK3β), as a drug that improves features of AC.[65] GSK3β is a negative regulator of canonical Wnt signaling, and inhibition of GSK3β activates this pathway. In this model, untreated mutant fish had defective protein trafficking in the intercalated discs in response to mutant plakoglobin. Subsequent treatment with SB216763 showed improvements in structural changes, arrhythmia, cardiac function, and survival. These data suggest a central role for GSK3β in the pathogenesis of AC.

The origin of adipocytes in AC has long been debated. To clarify the origin of these cells, experiments using lineage-tracing mice were designed.[66] By using genetic fate-mapping methods, the same group demonstrated that most of the adipocytes in AC originate from cardiac progenitor cells of the embryonic second heart field. Furthermore, in mice overexpressing cardiac truncated JUP, suppression of the canonical Wnt signaling pathway and induction of proadipogenic genes expression due to nuclear translocation of JUP led to adipogenesis in c-kit + cardiac progenitor cells.[67]

Moreover, a pathogenetic role of the Hippo/YAP signaling pathway has been identified. YAP interacts with β-catenin in the nucleus to drive Wnt-related gene expression. Chen and colleagues[68] demonstrated aberrant activation of the Hippo kinase cascade, resulting in phosphorylation and cytoplasmic retention of YAP; this causes β-catenin and JUP cytoplasmic sequestration, with further suppression of the canonical Wnt signaling leading to enhanced myocyte death and fibro-adipogenesis.

Patient-derived induced pluripotent stem cells (iPSCs) have enabled the generation of human cardiomyocytes for in vivo modeling. To this regard, Kim and colleagues,[69] by studying iPSCs-derived cardiomyocytes from AC patients with PKP2 mutations, demonstrated that the abnormal JUP nuclear translocation and decreased β-catenin activity are insufficient to reproduce the pathologic phenotype in standard conditions. Only the induction of an adultlike metabolism in a lipogenic milieu coactivated peroxisome proliferator-activated receptor-γ (PPAR-γ) pathway with lipogenesis, apoptosis, and calcium-handling deficit.

Noteworthy, experimental iPSC-derived cardiomyocytes demonstrated only abnormal "lipogenesis," but not adipocyte formation/transdifferentiation. Thus, cells other than cardiomyocytes must be involved in the abnormal adipogenesis and fibrosis, which are essential features of AC phenotype.[70] A role of cardiac mesenchymal stromal cells as a source of adipocytes in AC has been also suggested.[71]

Other mechanisms, such as epigenetic factors including microRNA, could contribute to desmosomal dysfunction and an AC phenotype and are currently under investigation.

Gap Junction and Ion Channel Remodeling

Desmosomes, gap junctions, and sodium channels act as a functional triad in which changes in the composition of one constituent can affect the function and integrity of the others.[4] Diminished expression of connexin-43 at the intercellular junction was demonstrated in most of the AC cases, suggesting that impaired mechanical coupling might also account for abnormal electrical coupling through gap-junction remodeling. Moreover, cardiac sodium current was found to be reduced in experimental models of AC.[29,72,73] These findings led to hypothesize that life-threatening ventricular arrhythmias could occur in AC patients, even preceding the structural abnormalities (prephenotypic stage) because of electrical uncoupling and reduced sodium current. However, this hypothesis remains to be proven in human AC patients, wherein only a reduced immunoreactive signal at intercalated disc for the major protein subunit of the sodium current Nav1.5 has been demonstrated.[73]

FUTURE PERSPECTIVES

The most important goals of clinical management of AC patients are sudden cardiac death prevention and improvement quality of life by decreasing or suppressing palpitations, VT recurrences, or ICD discharges.[12] Current therapeutic approaches, which are discussed in detail elsewhere and out of the scope of this review, regard lifestyle modifications, pharmacologic treatment, catheter ablation, ICD implantation, and exceptionally, heart transplantation. However, they are all palliative tools of symptomatic therapy, not addressing the disease onset and progression. It is hoped that ongoing experimental studies, by deciphering the signaling pathways of disease pathogenesis, together with a better understanding of environmental factors, will open the door to the identification of a targeted curative therapy in AC.

ACKNOWLEDGMENTS

This work has been supported by TRANSAC, University of Padua Strategic Grant CPDA133979/13, Padua, Italy; Registry for Cardio-Cerebro-Vascular Pathology, Veneto Region, Venice, Italy; Target Project, Regional Health System (RF-2014-00000394), Venice, Italy; PRIN Ministry of Education (2015ZLNETW), University and Research, Rome, Italy.

REFERENCES

1. Thiene G, Nava A, Corrado D, et al. Right ventricular cardiomyopathy and sudden death in young people. N Engl J Med 1988;318:129–33.
2. Basso C, Thiene G, Corrado D, et al. Arrhythmogenic right ventricular cardiomyopathy. Dysplasia,

dystrophy, or myocarditis? Circulation 1996;94:983–91.

3. Basso C, Corrado D, Marcus FI, et al. Arrhythmogenic right ventricular cardiomyopathy. Lancet 2009;373:1289–300.

4. Basso C, Bauce B, Corrado D, et al. Pathophysiology of arrhythmogenic cardiomyopathy. Nat Rev Cardiol 2011;9:223–33.

5. Nava A, Bauce B, Basso C, et al. Clinical profile and long-term follow-up of 37 families with arrhythmogenic right ventricular cardiomyopathy. J Am Coll Cardiol 2000;36:2226–33.

6. Corrado D, Basso C, Pavei A, et al. Trends in sudden cardiovascular death in young competitive athletes after implementation of a preparticipation screening program. JAMA 2006;296:1593–601.

7. Pilichou K, Thiene G, Bauce B, et al. Arrhythmogenic cardiomyopathy. Orphanet J Rare Dis 2016;11:33.

8. Basso C, Corrado D, Thiene G. Arrhythmogenic right ventricular cardiomyopathy: what's in a name? From a congenital defect (dysplasia) to a genetically determined cardiomyopathy (dystrophy). Am J Cardiol 2010;106:275–7.

9. Sen-Chowdhry S, Syrris P, Ward D, et al. Clinical and genetic characterization of families with arrhythmogenic right ventricular dysplasia/cardiomyopathy provides novel insights into patterns of disease expression. Circulation 2007;115:1710–20.

10. Thiene G, Nava A, Angelini A, et al. Anatomoclinical aspects of arrhythmogenic right ventricular cardiomyopathy. In: Baroldi G, Camerini F, Goodwin JF, editors. Advances in cardiomyopathies. Milan (Italy): Springer Verlag; 1990. p. 397–408.

11. Basso C, Corrado D, Bauce B, et al. Arrhythmogenic right ventricular cardiomyopathy. Circ Arrhythm Electrophysiol 2012;5:1233–46.

12. Corrado D, Wichter T, Link MS, et al. Treatment of arrhythmogenic right ventricular cardiomyopathy/dysplasia: an International Task Force Consensus statement. Circulation 2015;132:441–53.

13. Rizzo S, Lodder EM, Verkerk AO, et al. Intercalated disc abnormalities, reduced Na(+) current density, and conduction slowing in desmoglein-2 mutant mice prior to cardiomyopathic changes. Cardiovasc Res 2012;95:409–18.

14. Cerrone M, Noorman M, Lin X, et al. Sodium current deficit and arrhythmogenesis in a murine model of plakophilin-2 haploinsufficiency. Cardiovasc Res 2012;95:460–8.

15. McKenna WJ, Thiene G, Nava A, et al. Diagnosis of arrhythmogenic right ventricular dysplasia/cardiomyopathy. Task Force of the Working Group Myocardial and Pericardial Disease of the European Society of Cardiology and of the Scientific Council on Cardiomyopathies of the International Society and Federation of Cardiology. Br Heart J 1994;71:215–8.

16. Marcus FI, McKenna WJ, Sherrill D, et al. Diagnosis of arrhythmogenic right ventricular cardiomyopathy/dysplasia: proposed modification of the Task Force Criteria. Circulation 2010;121:1533–41.

17. Migliore F, Zorzi A, Michieli P, et al. Prevalence of cardiomyopathy in Italian asymptomatic children with electrocardiographic T-wave inversion at preparticipation screening. Circulation 2012;125:529–38.

18. Bauce B, Basso C, Rampazzo A, et al. Clinical profile of four families with arrhythmogenic right ventricular cardiomyopathy caused by dominant desmoplakin mutations. Eur Heart J 2005;26:1666–75.

19. Perazzolo Marra M, Leoni L, Bauce B, et al. Imaging study of ventricular scar in arrhythmogenic right ventricular cardiomyopathy: comparison of 3D standard electroanatomical voltage mapping and contrast-enhanced cardiac magnetic resonance. Circ Arrhythm Electrophysiol 2012;5:91–100.

20. Pilichou K, Mancini M, Rigato I, et al. Nonischemic left ventricular scar: sporadic or familial? Screen the genes, scan the mutation carriers. Circulation 2014;130:e180–2.

21. di Gioia CR, Giordano C, Cerbelli B, et al. Nonischemic left ventricular scar and cardiac sudden death in the young. Hum Pathol 2016;58:78–89.

22. Zorzi A, Perazzolo Marra M, Rigato I, et al. Nonischemic left ventricular scar as a substrate of life-threatening ventricular arrhythmias and sudden cardiac death in competitive athletes. Circ Arrhythm Electrophysiol 2016;9(7) [pii:e004229].

23. Basso C, Ronco F, Marcus F, et al. Quantitative assessment of endomyocardial biopsy in arrhythmogenic right ventricular cardiomyopathy/dysplasia: an in vitro validation of diagnostic criteria. Eur Heart J 2008;29:2760–71.

24. Corrado D, Basso C, Leoni L, et al. Three-dimensional electroanatomical voltage mapping and histologic evaluation of myocardial substrate in right ventricular outflow tract tachycardia. J Am Coll Cardiol 2008;51:731–9.

25. Migliore F, Zorzi A, Silvano M, et al. Prognostic value of endocardial voltage mapping in patients with arrhythmogenic right ventricular cardiomyopathy/dysplasia. Circ Arrhythm Electrophysiol 2013;6:167–76.

26. Garcia FC, Bazan V, Zado ES, et al. Epicardial substrate and outcome with epicardial ablation of ventricular tachycardia in arrhythmogenic right ventricular cardiomyopathy/dysplasia. Circulation 2009;120:366–75.

27. Zaidi A, Sharma S. Arrhythmogenic right ventricular remodelling in endurance athletes: Pandora's Box or Achilles' heel? Eur Heart J 2015;36(30):1955–7.

28. D'Ascenzi F, Pisicchio C, Caselli S, et al. RV remodeling in Olympic athletes. JACC Cardiovasc Imaging 2017;10(4):385–93.

29. Nava A, Thiene G, Canciani B, et al. Familial occurrence of right ventricular dysplasia: a study involving nine families. J Am Coll Cardiol 1988;12: 1222–8.

30. Protonotarios N, Tsatsopoulou A, Patsourakos P, et al. Cardiac abnormalities in familial palmoplantar keratosis. Br Heart J 1986;56:321–6.

31. McKoy G, Protonotarios N, Crosby A, et al. Identification of a deletion in plakoglobin in arrhythmogenic right ventricular cardiomyopathy with palmoplantar keratoderma and woolly hair (Naxos disease). Lancet 2000;355:2119–24.

32. Norgett EE, Hatsell SJ, Carvajal-Huerta L, et al. Recessive mutation in desmoplakin disrupts desmoplakin-intermediate filament interactions and causes dilated cardiomyopathy, woolly hair and keratoderma. Hum Mol Genet 2000;9:2761–6.

33. Rampazzo A, Nava A, Malacrida S, et al. Mutation in human desmoplakin domain binding to plakoglobin causes a dominant form of arrhythmogenic right ventricular cardiomyopathy. Am J Hum Genet 2002;71:1200–6.

34. Gerull B, Heuser A, Wichter T, et al. Mutations in the desmosomal protein plakophilin-2 are common in arrhythmogenic right ventricular cardiomyopathy. Nat Genet 2005;37:106.

35. Pilichou K, Nava A, Basso C, et al. Mutations in desmoglein-2 gene are associated with arrhythmogenic right ventricular cardiomyopathy. Circulation 2006;113:1171–9.

36. Syrris P, Ward D, Evans A, et al. Arrhythmogenic right ventricular dysplasia/cardiomyopathy associated with mutations in the desmosomal gene desmocollin-2. Am J Hum Genet 2006;79: 978–84.

37. Asimaki A, Syrris P, Wichter T, et al. A novel dominant mutation in plakoglobin causes arrhythmogenic right ventricular cardiomyopathy. Am J Hum Genet 2007;81:964–73.

38. Merner ND, Hodgkinson KA, Haywood AF, et al. Arrhythmogenic right ventricular cardiomyopathy type 5 is a fully penetrant, lethal arrhythmic disorder caused by a missense mutation in the TMEM43 gene. Am J Hum Genet 2008;82:809–21.

39. van Tintelen JP, Van Gelder IC, Asimaki A, et al. Severe cardiac phenotype with right ventricular predominance in a large cohort of patients with a single missense mutation in the DES gene. Heart Rhythm 2009;6:1574–83.

40. van der Zwaag PA, Cox MG, van der Werf C, et al. Plakophilin-2 p.Arg79X mutation causing arrhythmogenic right ventricular cardiomyopathy/dysplasia. Neth Heart J 2010;18:583–91.

41. Taylor M, Graw S, Sinagra G, et al. Genetic variation in titin in arrhythmogenic right ventricular cardiomyopathy-overlap syndromes. Circulation 2011;124:876–85.

42. Quarta G, Syrris P, Ashworth M, et al. Mutations in the lamin A/C gene mimic arrhythmogenic right ventricular cardiomyopathy. Eur Heart J 2012;33: 1128–36.

43. van Hengel J, Calore M, Bauce B, et al. Mutations in the area composita protein αT-catenin are associated with arrhythmogenic right ventricular cardiomyopathy. Eur Heart J 2013;34:201–10.

44. Ortiz-Genga MF, Cuenca S, Dal Ferro M, et al. Truncating FLNC mutations are associated with high-risk dilated and arrhythmogenic cardiomyopathies. J Am Coll Cardiol 2016;68:2440–51.

45. Mayosi BM, Fish M, Shaboodien G, et al. Identification of cadherin 2 (CDH2) mutations in arrhythmogenic right ventricular cardiomyopathy. Circ Cardiovasc Genet 2017;10 [pii:e001605].

46. Beffagna G, Occhi G, Nava A, et al. Regulatory mutations in transforming growth factor-beta3 gene cause arrhythmogenic right ventricular cardiomyopathy type 1. Cardiovasc Res 2005; 65:366–73.

47. Franke WW, Borrmann CM, Grund C, et al. The area composita of adhering junctions connecting heart muscle cells of vertebrates. I. Molecular definition in intercalated disks of cardiomyocytes by immunoelectron microscopy of desmosomal proteins. Eur J Cell Biol 2006;85:69–82.

48. Bauce B, Nava A, Beffagna G, et al. Multiple mutations in desmosomal proteins encoding genes in arrhythmogenic right ventricular cardiomyopathy/dysplasia. Heart Rhythm 2010;7:22–9.

49. Rigato I, Bauce B, Rampazzo A, et al. Compound and digenic heterozygosity predicts lifetime arrhythmic outcome and sudden cardiac death in desmosomal gene-related arrhythmogenic right ventricular cardiomyopathy. Circ Cardiovasc Genet 2013;6:533–42.

50. Xu T, Yang Z, Vatta M, et al, Multidisciplinary Study of Right Ventricular Dysplasia Investigators. Compound and digenic heterozygosity contributes to arrhythmogenic right ventricular cardiomyopathy. J Am Coll Cardiol 2010;55:587–97.

51. Lazzarini E, Jongbloed JD, Pilichou K, et al. The ARVD/C genetic variants database: 2014 update. Hum Mutat 2015;36:403–10.

52. Bhonsale A, Groeneweg JA, James CA, et al. Impact of genotype on clinical course in arrhythmogenic right ventricular dysplasia/cardiomyopathy-associated mutation carriers. Eur Heart J 2015;36: 847–55.

53. Cox MG, van der Zwaag PA, van der Werf C, et al. Arrhythmogenic right ventricular dysplasia/cardiomyopathy: pathogenic desmosome mutations in index-patients predict outcome of family screening: Dutch arrhythmogenic right ventricular dysplasia/cardiomyopathy genotype-phenotype follow-up study. Circulation 2011;123:2690–700.

54. Pilichou K, Lazzarini E, Rigato I, et al. Large genomic rearrangements of desmosomal genes in italian arrhythmogenic cardiomyopathy patients. Circ Arrhythm Electrophysiol 2017;10(10) [pii: e005324].

55. Dalal D, James C, Devanagondi R, et al. Penetrance of mutations in plakophilin-2 among families with arrhythmogenic right ventricular dysplasia/cardiomyopathy. J Am Coll Cardiol 2006;48:1416–24.

56. van Tintelen JP, Entius MM, Bhuiyan ZA, et al. Plakophilin-2 mutations are the major determinant of familial arrhythmogenic right ventricular dysplasia/cardiomyopathy. Circulation 2006;113:1650–8.

57. Norman M, Simpson M, Mogensen J, et al. Novel mutation in desmoplakin causes arrhythmogenic left ventricular cardiomyopathy. Circulation 2005; 112(5):636–42.

58. Quarta G, Muir A, Pantazis A, et al. Familial evaluation in arrhythmogenic right ventricular cardiomyopathy: impact of genetics and revised task force criteria. Circulation 2011;123:2701–9.

59. Fressart V, Duthoit G, Donal E, et al. Desmosomal gene analysis in arrhythmogenic right ventricular dysplasia/cardiomyopathy: spectrum of mutations and clinical impact in practice. Europace 2010;12: 861–8.

60. Corrado D, Basso C, Judge DP. Arrhythmogenic cardiomyopathy. Circ Res 2017;121(7):784–802.

61. Pilichou K, Remme CA, Basso C, et al. Myocyte necrosis underlies progressive myocardial dystrophy in mouse dsg2-related arrhythmogenic right ventricular cardiomyopathy. J Exp Med 2009;206: 1787–802.

62. Basso C, Czarnowska E, Della Barbera M, et al. Ultrastructural evidence of intercalated disc remodelling in arrhythmogenic right ventricular cardiomyopathy: an electron microscopy investigation on endomyocardial biopsies. Eur Heart J 2006;27: 1847–54.

63. Garcia-Gras E, Lombardi R, Giocondo MJ, et al. Suppression of canonical Wnt/beta-catenin signaling by nuclear plakoglobin recapitulates phenotype of arrhythmogenic right ventricular cardiomyopathy. J Clin Invest 2006;116:2012–21.

64. Lombardi R, Dong J, Rodriguez G, et al. Genetic fate mapping identifies second heart field progenitor cells as a source of adipocytes in arrhythmogenic right ventricular cardiomyopathy. Circ Res 2009; 104:1076–84.

65. James CA, Bhonsale A, Tichnell C, et al. Exercise increases age-related penetrance and arrhythmic risk in arrhythmogenic right ventricular dysplasia/cardiomyopathy-associated desmosomal mutation carriers. J Am Coll Cardiol 2013;62:1290–7.

66. Asimaki A, Kapoor S, Plovie E, et al. Identification of a new modulator of the intercalated disc in a zebrafish model of arrhythmogenic cardiomyopathy. Sci Transl Med 2014;6:240ra74.

67. Lombardi R, da Graca Cabreira-Hansen M, Bell A, et al. Nuclear plakoglobin is essential for differentiation of cardiac progenitor cells to adipocytes in arrhythmogenic right ventricular cardiomyopathy. Circ Res 2011;109:1342–53.

68. Chen SN, Gurha P, Lombardi R, et al. The hippo pathway is activated and is a causal mechanism for adipogenesis in arrhythmogenic cardiomyopathy. Circ Res 2014;114:454–68.

69. Kim C, Wong J, Wen J, et al. Studying arrhythmogenic right ventricular dysplasia with patient-specific iPSCs. Nature 2013;494:105–10.

70. Wen JY, Wei CY, Shah K, et al. Maturation-based model of arrhythmogenic right ventricular dysplasia using patient-specific induced pluripotent stem cells. Circ J 2015;79:1402–8.

71. Sommariva E, Brambilla S, Carbucicchio C, et al. Cardiac mesenchymal stromal cells are a source of adipocytes in arrhythmogenic cardiomyopathy. Eur Heart J 2016;37(23):1835–46.

72. Zhang Q, Deng C, Rao F, et al. Silencing of desmoplakin decreases connexin43/Nav1.5 expression and sodium current in HL-1 cardiomyocytes. Mol Med Rep 2013;8:780–6.

73. Noorman M, Hakim S, Kessler E, et al. Remodeling of the cardiac sodium channel, connexin43, and plakoglobin at the intercalated disk in patients with arrhythmogenic cardiomyopathy. Heart Rhythm 2013; 10:412–9.

Genetic Infiltrative Cardiomyopathies

Mary E. Sweet, BA, Luisa Mestroni, MD, Matthew R.G. Taylor, MD, PhD*

KEYWORDS

- Amyloidosis • Hemochromatosis • Cardiac oxalosis • Friedreich ataxia • Mucopolysaccharidosis
- Fabry disease • Danon disease • PRKAG2 syndrome

KEY POINTS

- Infiltrative cardiomyopathies result from progressive buildup of abnormal substances in the heart.
- Several infiltrative cardiomyopathies are inherited and have known genetic mechanisms.
- Each inherited infiltrative cardiomyopathy has distinct extracardiac manifestations.
- Although the pathologic mechanisms, type of infiltrative substances, and extracardiac presentations differ, many of these cardiomyopathies have similar or overlapping cardiac presentations.

INTRODUCTION

Infiltrative cardiomyopathies are characterized by abnormal deposition or accumulation of substances in the heart. Essentially, these diseases have similarities and overlaps in echocardiographic and cardiovascular presentation, but they display a broad range of seemingly disparate extracardiac features. This review article specifically discusses the inherited infiltrative cardiomyopathies, giving an overview of the genes, molecular mechanisms, and resulting features of each disease, with emphasis on the heart. **Fig. 1** summarizes the cellular mechanisms and phenotypes and **Table 1** summarizes the genetic features of each disease.

This review begins with the extracardiac diseases that primarily manifest in other organs and only reach the heart through substance accumulation in the bloodstream. Then it moves on to the intracardiac diseases that can manifest directly within the cardiac myocytes.

EXTRACARDIAC INFILTRATIVE CARDIOMYOPATHIES
Transthyretin Cardiac Amyloidosis

Amyloidosis is a general term for extracellular accumulation of amyloids, or protein aggregates, that form ß-pleated fibrous deposits. Amyloidosis can be acquired or inherited and can present with multiorgan involvement. For the purposes of this review, only the inherited form is discussed. Inherited amyloidosis is caused by mutations in *TTR*, which encodes transthyretin, a serum and cerebrospinal fluid transport protein secreted almost exclusively (>98%) by the liver.[1] TTR transports thyroxine and retinol, from which it gets its name. Point mutations in *TTR* can destabilize the tetramer, increasing the likelihood that it will disassociate into amyloidogenic monomers, aggregate into fibrils, and deposit into organs. Progressive deposition of amyloid in the heart can lead to cardiac amyloidosis.

Transthyretin cardiac amyloidosis is inherited in an autosomal dominant manner. Although some

Disclosures: There are no conflicts of interest or financial disclosures associated with this work.
Adult Medical Genetics Program, Cardiovascular Institute, University of Colorado Anschutz, 12700 East 19th Avenue, Aurora, CO 80045, USA
* Corresponding author. Adult Medical Genetics Program, University of Colorado Denver, 12700 East 19th Avenue, F442, Room 8022, Aurora, CO 80045.
E-mail address: matthew.taylor@ucdenver.edu

heartfailure.theclinics.com

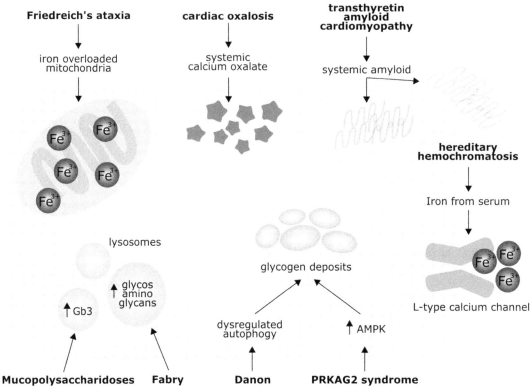

Fig. 1. Genetic infiltrative cardiomyopathy in the cardiac myocyte. AMPK, adenosine monophosphate–activated protein kinase; Gb3, globotriaosylceramide.

TTR mutations present with predictable phenotypes, affecting predominately the heart or liver, most genotype–phenotype correlations in *TTR* have unpredictable prognoses[2] due in part to the contribution of noncoding variation in *TTR* regulation. Noncoding variation in *TTR* that affects TTR tissue-specific expression identifies clusters of TTR amyloid patients with similar phenotypes. This suggests that complex genetics contributes to the variable expressivity of TTR amyloidosis.[3] The most frequent variant in TTR amyloid is *TTR* p.V122I, which had reported throughout the literature to be present in 3% to 4% of African Americans, though it is only present in 1.6% of the African population within the Genome Aggregation Database (gnomAD).[4,5] In a recent study of 156 African Americans referred for amyloidosis, the *TTR* V122I (V142I) mutation was present in 23%, and most of these subjects developed *TTR* amyloidosis.[6]

Pathogenic mutations in *TTR* are primarily clinically characterized by progressive neuropathy (86% of cases) or cardiomyopathy (42% of cases) with some overlap.[7] Cardiomyopathy presents on average in the fourth decade of life but can range significantly from less than 20 years to greater than 80 years.[7] Cardiac amyloidosis typically presents as heart failure with preserved ejection fraction.[8]

Historically, the standard treatment of transthyretin cardiac amyloidosis has been liver transplantation, sometimes in combination with heart transplantation. However, several therapies are being developed or are in clinical trials that stabilize TTR tetramers (tafamidis, diflunisal, AG10), degrade preexisting amyloid deposits (doxycycline, anti-serum amyloid protein P [SAP]), or silence transthyretin protein production (RNA interference [RNAi]).[9] Stabilizers bind to the TTR tetramer and prevent its disassociation, but the selectivity of the compounds and their ability to effectively bind various pathogenic variants of TTR are issues to consider. Degraders target amyloid protein that has already been deposited. For example, SAP is a universal constituent of amyloid protein; targeting SAP with an antibody significantly reduces amyloid deposits in animal models.[10,11] Finally, silencing amyloid protein production is also a potential therapy. The largest randomized phase 3 trial to date in hereditary transthyretin amyloidosis is currently underway, using RNAi technology to target a conserved messenger RNA (mRNA) sequence across both wildtype and mutated TTR transcripts. The

Table 1
Summary of the genetics of inherited cardiomyopathies

Inherited Infiltrative Cardiomyopathy	Disease Type	Infiltrative Substance	Modes of Inheritance	Genes
Extracardiac				
Transthyretin cardiac amyloidosis	Amyloidosis	Amyloid	Autosomal dominant	TTR
Hereditary hemochromatosis	Disease of iron metabolism	Iron	Autosomal recessive (types 1–3); autosomal dominant (type 4)	HFE (type 1), HJV, HAMP (type 2), TFR2 (type 3), SLC40A1 (type 4)
Cardiac oxalosis	Disease of glyoxylate metabolism	Calcium oxalate	Autosomal recessive	AGXT (type 1), GRHPR (type 2), HOGA1 (type 3)
Intracardiac				
Friedreich ataxia	Disease of iron metabolism	Iron	Autosomal recessive	FXN
Mucopolysaccharidoses	Lysosomal storage disease	Glycosaminoglycans	Autosomal recessive (I, III, IV, VI, VII, IX); X-linked recessive (II)	IDUA (I), IDS (II), SGSH, NAGLU, HGSNAT, GNS (III), GALNS, GLB1 (IV), ARSB (VI), GUSB (VII), HYAL1 (IX)
Fabry disease	Lysosomal storage disease	Globotriaosylceramide	X-linked	GLA
Danon disease	Disease of autophagy	Glycogen	X-linked	LAMP2
PRKAG2 syndrome	Glycogen storage disease	Glycogen	Autosomal dominant	PRKAG2

small interfering RNA (siRNA) is directed to the liver with the goal of suppressing TTR hepatic production and reducing circulating levels of the protein.[12,13]

Hereditary Hemochromatosis

Hemochromatosis is a progressive condition of iron accumulation and end-organ damage. Hemochromatosis is caused by mutations in genes encoding proteins involved in iron absorption, transportation, and storage. There are 4 types caused by mutations in their corresponding genes: type 1, *HFE*; type 2, *HAMP* or *HJV*; type 3, *TFR2*; and type 4, *SLC40A1*. Types I, 3, and 4, are adult-onset diseases and present in the fourth to fifth decade of life; in contrast, type 2 is a juvenile-onset disease and presents in the second or third decade. Hereditary hemochromatosis is inherited as an autosomal recessive trait, except type 4, which is autosomal dominant.[14]

By far the most common genotype risk for hereditary hemochromatosis is *HFE* p.Cys282Tyr homozygosity, which accounts for more than 80% of patients.[15] The mutation that causes p.Cys282Tyr is heterozygous in 1 per 9 non-Finnish Europeans and homozygous in 1 per 538, according to gnomAD.[16] However, depending on the geographic region, the frequency, even within Europeans, can vary.[15] It is also present in lower frequencies in all other ethnicities, with the lowest frequencies in South and East Asian populations.[16] Homozygosity for p.Cys282Tyr demonstrates incomplete penetrance; it causes hemochromatosis in 1% to 14% of female patients and 24% to 28% of male patients.[17,18] This difference is attributed in part to recurrent physiologic blood loss in women that contributes to slower iron accumulation[18] but may result from other genetic or environmental factors.

Due to the heterogeneous phenotypic expression of the pC282Y/pC282Y genotype,[18] it has been hypothesized that additional genetic modifiers played a role. In patients homozygous for p.Cys282Tyr, heterozygous missense or loss-of-function mutations in *HJV* or *HAMP* contribute to a more severe iron overload.[19,20] Additionally, a combination of heterozygous missense mutations in *HAMP* and *HFE* can also cause hemochromatosis.[19] Although *HFE* causal genotypes lead to adult-onset hemochromatosis, homozygous loss-of-function in *HAMP*[21] and homozygous missense mutations in *HJV*[22] can cause juvenile-onset hereditary hemochromatosis.

The iron overload that results from hemochromatosis can cause dilated or restrictive cardiomyopathy[14] and can manifest with conduction abnormalities and tachyarrhythmia.[14] During iron overload, L-type calcium channels in cardiomyocytes can uptake excess iron, which elicits harmful free radical production in the cell.[23] Calcium channel blockers have been used effectively in mice to decrease cardiac iron accumulation but have not been studied in humans.[24,25] Cellular injury from iron overload-induced free radical production may be exacerbated in patients receiving doxorubicin chemotherapy, due to formation of doxorubicin-iron complexes in the mitochondria.[26,27] This can lead to increased risk of doxorubicin-induced cardiotoxicity in hemochromatosis patients, resulting in diastolic dysfunction.[26,28] Therapy for hereditary hemochromatosis includes cardiac transplantation,[29] phlebotomy, and iron chelation.[30]

Cardiac Oxalosis

Primary hyperoxaluria (PH) is an autosomal recessive disease of glyoxylate metabolism that causes oxalate overproduction. PH is divided into 3 types, each caused by mutations in different genes that encode enzymes involved in glyoxylate metabolism: type I, alanine-glyoxylate aminotransferase (*AGXT*); type II, glyoxylate reductase/hydroxypyruvate reductase (*GRHPR*); type III, 4-hydroxy-2-oxoglutarate aldolase (*HOGA1*). PH type 1, which accounts for almost 80% of all cases,[31] has a prevalence of 1 to 3 per 1 million people.[32,33]

In PH, glyoxylate accumulates and is converted to oxalate, which cannot be metabolized. Recurrent urolithiasis and progressive nephrocalcinosis lead to kidney damage, consequent reductions in excreted oxalate, increased systemic levels of oxalate, and subsequent calcium oxalate deposition in tissues.[34] The organs affected include skin, bone, the retina, vessels, and the myocardium.[35]

After the kidneys become damaged and oxalate begins to deposit in the tissues, it often results in end-stage renal disease, but cardiac symptoms can also occur. However, PH is an extremely rare disease and not all patients experience cardiac dysfunction. In a review study of cardiac phenotypes in 38 PH subjects, approximately 11% experienced dyspnea, 9% experienced chest pain and palpitation, and 3% experienced syncope. The most common echocardiographic findings were increased left ventricular mass (29%) and left atrium enlargement (21%), and abnormal electrocardiogram findings included left ventricular hypertrophy (5%), bundle branch block (9%), and atrioventricular block (5%).[36] There have also been reports of PH patients presenting with ventricular tachycardia,[37] mitral valve regurgitation,[38] restrictive cardiomyopathy[39] and heart failure.[38] Combined liver and kidney transplantation has been shown to reverse cardiac dysfunction and oxalate deposits in the heart.[40]

INTRACARDIAC INFILTRATIVE CARDIOMYOPATHIES
Friedreich Ataxia

Friedreich ataxia is primarily a neurodegenerative disorder but is also characterized by other multisystemic effects. Progressive neurologic features include poor balance, muscle weakness, loss of motor skills, and visual and hearing impairment. Other nonneurological complications include scoliosis, diabetes mellitus, and hypertrophic cardiomyopathy (HCM).[41]

Friedreich ataxia is autosomal recessive with an estimated prevalence of 3 to 4 per 100,000.[42] It is caused by unstable expansion of a trinucleotide repeat in the first intron of *FXN* that inhibits transcription elongation. Repeats in the nascent transcript form tertiary structures, called R-loops, with the genomic DNA, leading to reduced expression.[43,44] *FXN* encodes frataxin, a mitochondrial protein involved in iron homeostasis. Frataxin deficiency is associated with dysregulated iron trafficking leading to mitochondrial iron aggregation.[45–48] Unaffected persons typically have less than 12 repeats, but they can range from 12 to 59.[42] Friedreich ataxia patients have 60 to 1500.[41] Whereas 97% of patients are homozygous for this expansion,[41] the remaining individuals are compound heterozygous; on 1 allele they have the expansion and on the other a loss-of-function point mutation.[41,49] All reported patients have at least 1 expanded allele, and animal models suggest that homozygous loss-of-function is embryonic lethal.[50]

The age of onset can range significantly, from less than 1 year to 70 years, with a mean age of 12 to 16 years and a mean age of death of 37 years.[41,51] Young age of onset, disease severity, and degree of diastolic dysfunction are generally predicted by higher numbers of trinucleotide repeats.[41,51,52] However, the age of onset only accounts for 36% of the variability in trinucleotide repeats, suggesting additional genetic modifiers may play a role.[41] One study, for example, showed that *FXN* methylation can predict frataxin expression and clinical outcome.[53]

Although cardiomyopathy is the presenting finding in only 5% of patients,[41] cardiac dysfunction from congestive heart failure or arrhythmia accounts for an estimated 59% of death.[51] Individuals with homozygous expansions are more likely to develop cardiomyopathy.[53] Cardiac dysfunction includes left ventricular hypertrophy,

systolic dysfunction, and diastolic dysfunction.[52] Current treatment options that address the cardiac issues in Friedreich ataxia are limited to antioxidants; iron chelation; and, uncommonly, cardiac transplantation in patients with heart failure.[46,54] Many reports of antioxidant treatment[42] or combined antioxidant and iron chelation[55] decreased left ventricular mass and improved cardiac function, but other studies have found no changes after therapy.[56]

Mucopolysaccharidoses

Mucopolysaccharidoses (MPS) is a group of lysosomal storage disorders that result from deficient glycosaminoglycan-degrading enzymes. Glycosaminoglycans build up in the lysosomes of cells, leading to progressive tissue and organ dysfunction. Deficiency in 11 different enzymes is known to cause 7 different MPS phenotypes that are inherited in either an autosomal recessive (MPS I, III, IV, VI, VII, IX) or X-linked recessive (MPS II) fashion. There are also several reported cases in which MPS II has occurred in female patients via skewed lionization.[57–59]

MPS are quite rare, with an overall prevalence of 1 per 22,000.[60] Among these, MPS 1, among the relatively more common MPS, has a reported prevalence of 1 per 35,000.[61] Depending on the phenotype and the degree of enzyme deficiency, typical life expectancy can range from infancy to the fifth decade. Cardiac abnormalities have been reported for all MPS types, particularly I, II, and IV, and occur in most of the subjects studied (60%–100%, depending on the study).[62] The most common cardiac phenotypes in MPS are hypertrophy and valve disease. In MPS I, II, and VI, 50% of patients have increased left ventricular mass due to either concentric (I and II) or eccentric hypertrophy (VI). Approximately 50% to 60% of patients have valvular regurgitation in at least 1 valve, and all patients have abnormal valves. Valve replacement in MPS is common but can be challenging given concomitant respiratory compromise seen in many MPS patients.[63,64] Impaired systolic function is less common but present.[65,66] Other MPS VI patients have experienced sinus tachycardia, left atrial dilation, and congestive heart failure.[16,66]

Intravenous enzyme replacement therapy is a strategy to treat MPS and is currently available for MPS I, II, and VI. Due to its progressive nature, early enzyme replacement therapy may stabilize or slow disease progression, including cardiac dysfunction, and sibling control studies have suggested that the earlier the intervention, the better.[67,68] Therapy decreased left ventricular mass in MPS I, II, and VI,[65] and decreased intraventricular septal hypertrophy in MPS VI,[69] but it did not affect physiologic valvular regurgitation.[65,69] Another study in MPS VI showed stabilization but not improvement of cardiac function.[70]

Fabry Disease

Similar to the MPS, Fabry disease is also a lysosomal storage disorder, but it results in progressive accumulation of a type of fat, particularly globotriaosylceramide (Gb3), in lysosomes. Fabry disease is an X-linked trait resulting from partial or complete deficiency of α-galactosidase A, a lysosomal enzyme encoded by *GLA*. Due to the ubiquitous nature of lysosomes, Fabry results in progressive dysfunction of multiple organs, including the kidneys, brain, and heart. Enzyme activity is inversely related to both age of onset and disease severity; some variants that maintain 2% to 20% enzymatic function result in attenuated phenotypes that present much later in life with fewer symptoms.[71,72] Typically, female heterozygotes present with a milder form of the disease and later in life than male patients, but severity of symptoms may increase with skewed lyonization.[73]

Historically, the prevalence estimates for Fabry have suggested it is a relatively rare disease; however, the newest estimates, based on recent newborn screening data, suggest it is more common than previously thought.[72] Typically, the newborn screening process will assay α-galactosidase A enzyme activity in blood spots followed by confirmatory genetic testing. Results from these studies support a prevalence ranging approximately 1 per 1400 to 7800 in male patients.[61,74,75]

Typically, Fabry disease presents in early childhood with an array of symptoms, including hypohidrosis (reduced or absent sweating); autonomic nervous system dysfunction, leading to gastrointestinal issues; and acroparesthesia pains in the extremities, especially in the setting of viral illnesses or fevers.[72,76] They can also present in childhood with cardiac findings. The most common are increased left ventricular mass and valvular dysfunction, but reduced heart rate variability and electrocardiograph changes such as T-wave inversion and PR prolongation can also occur.[76–78] Nonclassical Fabry disease is more variable and may manifest only with cardiac dysfunction.[71] As children with Fabry disease age, their cardiac manifestations progress into more severe cardiac problems, including hypertrophic or dilated cardiomyopathy phenotype, arrhythmia, heart failure, and sudden cardiac death.[79,80] Fabry disease may be responsible for 12% of late-onset HCM in female patients,

suggesting that the condition may be underreported in female patients.[81] Enzyme replacement therapy is clinically available for these patients and, although not able to cure Fabry disease, it has been shown to slow disease progression in some studies, particularly when administered at an earlier stage.[82–85]

Danon

Danon disease is an X-linked dominant disease that predominantly affects the heart but is also characterized by skeletal myopathy and intellectual disability. Danon is caused by mutations in *LAMP2*, which encodes the lysosome-associated membrane glycoprotein 2. The earliest histopathological studies of muscle biopsies from Danon subjects demonstrated glycogen deposits in lysosomes, leading to the conclusion that it was primarily a glycogen storage disease.[86] However, continued genetic and cellular studies have suggested that it is instead a disease of deficient autophagy that leads to glycogen accumulation.[87,88]

LAMP2 encodes 3 isoforms via differential splicing, with LAMP2-A and LAMP2-B significantly more expressed than LAMP2-C in the heart.[88] Although most described mutations in *LAMP2* affect all 3 isoforms, there are reports of mutations that only affect the LAMP2-B isoform, suggesting that deficiency of this isoform is necessary and sufficient to cause disease.[87,88] For a complete review of the molecular biology of *LAMP2* in Danon, see the recent review by Rowland and colleagues[88] (2016). Generally, loss-of-function mutations are associated with an earlier age of onset compared with missense mutations.[87] Due to homozygosity and skewed X-inactivation, Danon affects male patients earlier and more severely than female patients. Male patients typically experience first symptom, cardiac transplantation, and death at ages 12, 18, and 19, respectively. These experiences are delayed approximately 15 years in female patients who manifest the disease.[89–91]

Danon disease primarily affects the heart. Male patients present more often with hypertrophy (HCM phenotype) and female patients with dilation (dilated cardiomyopathy phenotype).[89,90] Cardiomyopathy manifests as left ventricular systolic dysfunction; ventricular preexcitation associated with T-wave inversion; palpitations; conduction abnormalities and Wolff-Parkinson-White syndrome; and rapid, progressive heart failure, resulting in transplantation or death.[89,91,92] Although there are no specific evidence-driven guidelines for management of Danon, there are published recommendations. Due to the rapid, progressive nature of Danon, early monitoring of electrophysiology and early consideration of implantable cardioverter-defibrillator (ICD) implantation is suggested, particularly in patients with symptomatic arrhythmias, moderate to severe hypertrophy, fibrosis, or a positive family history for sudden cardiac death.[87] The molecular mechanism by which defective or deficient *LAMP2* causes Danon remains elusive, but activation of autophagy via activation of the Akt-mTORC1 pathway has been an effective therapy in a mouse model of HCM, and may be a potential target for Danon.[93]

PRKAG2 Syndrome

Like Danon, PRKAG2 syndrome also results in the accumulation of glycogen in the cardiomyocyte. *PRKAG2* encodes the gamma-2 subunit of adenosine monophosphate–activated protein kinase (AMPK). AMPK is a cellular fuel gauge that is constantly sensing and responding to the energy needs of the cell, particularly in cardiomyocyte metabolism.[94] PRKAG2 syndrome is inherited in an autosomal dominant manner with high penetrance. Mutations in *PRKAG2* alter the binding affinity and enzymatic activity of AMPK, activating AMPK activity and glycogen accumulation.[95] Pathologic analysis of human tissue from patients with *PRKAG2* mutations suggests that cardiac hypertrophy and conduction system disease are the manifesting symptoms of a glycogen storage disease. Patient tissue demonstrated myocyte enlargement and minimal interstitial fibrosis, consistent with hypertrophy, but also revealed the presence of vacuoles containing glycogen-derivatives within myocytes.[96]

Clinically, PRKAG2 syndrome leads to cardiac hypertrophy, supraventricular arrhythmias, and conduction abnormalities such as preexcitation, particularly in the context of Wolff-Parkinson-White Syndrome.[97] Patients often present with palpitations and syncope.[98] Reports indicating the onset of PRKAG2 syndrome range widely from infantile-fatal to the fifth decade of life with a mean age of onset of 30 years,[92,99,100] though an infantile-fatal mutation has been reported.[100] Similar to Danon, there are no specific guidelines for PRKAG2 syndrome; however, suggested guidelines include assessment of risk factors for sudden death (symptomatic arrhythmias, family history) and early consideration for pacemaker or ICD implantation.[99] Because AMPK is activated in PRKAG2 syndrome, a small molecule inhibitor of AMPK may be an effective therapy, but this has not been tested.

SUMMARY

The genetic infiltrative cardiomyopathies have overlapping presentations in the heart but are characterized by a diversity of diseases. These diseases manifest in multisystemic mechanisms with cardiomyopathy as either a primary or secondary feature. Each disease has distinct genes and mechanisms, but can adversely affect the heart in similar ways.

REFERENCES

1. Lachmann HJ. A new era in the treatment of amyloidosis? N Engl J Med 2013;369(9):866–8.
2. Zeldenrust SR. Genotype–phenotype correlation in FAP. Amyloid 2012;19(Suppl 1):22–4.
3. Iorio A, De Lillo A, De Angelis F, et al. Non-coding variants contribute to the clinical heterogeneity of TTR amyloidosis. Eur J Hum Genet 2017;25(9): 1055–60.
4. Schneider JL, Cuervo AM. Autophagy and human disease: emerging themes. Curr Opin Genet Dev 2014;26:16–23.
5. Jacobson DR, Pastore RD, Yaghoubian R, et al. Variant-sequence transthyretin (isoleucine 122) in late-onset cardiac amyloidosis in black Americans. N Engl J Med 1997;336(7):466–73.
6. Connors LH, Prokaeva T, Lim A, et al. Cardiac amyloidosis in African Americans: comparison of clinical and laboratory features of transthyretin V122I amyloidosis and immunoglobulin light chain amyloidosis. Am Heart J 2009;158(4): 607–14.
7. Coelho T, Maurer MS, Suhr OB. THAOS - The Transthyretin Amyloidosis Outcomes Survey: initial report on clinical manifestations in patients with hereditary and wild-type transthyretin amyloidosis. Curr Med Res Opin 2013;29(1): 63–76.
8. Mohammed SF, Mirzoyev SA, Edwards WD, et al. Left ventricular amyloid deposition in patients with heart failure and preserved ejection fraction. JACC Heart Fail 2014;2(2):113–22.
9. Castano A, Drachman BM, Judge D, et al. Natural history and therapy of TTR-cardiac amyloidosis: emerging disease-modifying therapies from organ transplantation to stabilizer and silencer drugs. Heart Fail Rev 2015;20(2):163–78.
10. Bodin K, Ellmerich S, Kahan MC, et al. Antibodies to human serum amyloid P component eliminate visceral amyloid deposits. Nature 2010;468(7320):93–7.
11. Pepys MB, Herbert J, Hutchinson WL, et al. Targeted pharmacological depletion of serum amyloid P component for treatment of human amyloidosis. Nature 2002;417(6886):254–9.

12. Coelho T, Adams D, Silva A, et al. Safety and efficacy of RNAi therapy for transthyretin amyloidosis. New Engl J Med 2013;369(9):819–29.

13. Adams D, Suhr OB, Dyck PJ, et al. Trial design and rationale for APOLLO, a Phase 3, placebo-controlled study of patisiran in patients with hereditary ATTR amyloidosis with polyneuropathy. BMC Neurol 2017;17(1):181.

14. Kremastinos DT, Farmakis D. Iron overload cardiomyopathy in clinical practice. Circulation 2011;124(20):2253–63.

15. European Association for the Study of the Liver. EASL clinical practice guidelines for HFE hemochromatosis. J Hepatol 2010;53(1):3–22.

16. Azevedo AC, Schwartz IV, Kalakun L, et al. Clinical and biochemical study of 28 patients with mucopolysaccharidosis type VI. Clin Genet 2004;66(3):208–13.

17. Gallego CJ, Burt A, Sundaresan AS, et al. Penetrance of Hemochromatosis in HFE Genotypes Resulting in p.Cys282Tyr and p.[Cys282Tyr];[His63Asp] in the eMERGE network. Am J Hum Genet 2015;97(4):512–20.

18. Allen KJ, Gurrin LC, Constantine CC, et al. Iron-overload-related disease in HFE hereditary hemochromatosis. New Engl J Med 2008;358(3):221–30.

19. Jacolot S, Le Gac G, Scotet V, et al. HAMP as a modifier gene that increases the phenotypic expression of the HFE pC282Y homozygous genotype. Blood 2004;103(7):2835–40.

20. Le Gac G, Scotet V, Ka C, et al. The recently identified type 2A juvenile haemochromatosis gene (HJV), a second candidate modifier of the C282Y homozygous phenotype. Hum Mol Genet 2004;13(17):1913–8.

21. Roetto A, Papanikolaou G, Politou M, et al. Mutant antimicrobial peptide hepcidin is associated with severe juvenile hemochromatosis. Nat Genet 2003;33(1):21–2.

22. Papanikolaou G, Samuels ME, Ludwig EH, et al. Mutations in HFE2 cause iron overload in chromosome 1q-linked juvenile hemochromatosis. Nat Genet 2004;36(1):77–82.

23. Tsushima RG, Wickenden AD, Bouchard RA, et al. Modulation of iron uptake in heart by L-type Ca2+ channel modifiers: possible implications in iron overload. Circ Res 1999;84(11):1302–9.

24. Oudit GY, Sun H, Trivieri MG, et al. L-type Ca2+ channels provide a major pathway for iron entry into cardiomyocytes in iron-overload cardiomyopathy. Nat Med 2003;9(9):1187–94.

25. Ludwiczek S, Theurl I, Muckenthaler MU, et al. Ca2+ channel blockers reverse iron overload by a new mechanism via divalent metal transporter-1. Nat Med 2007;13(4):448–54.

26. Lipshultz SE, Lipsitz SR, Kutok JL, et al. Impact of hemochromatosis gene mutations on cardiac status in doxorubicin-treated survivors of childhood high-risk leukemia. Cancer 2013;119(19):3555–62.

27. Panjrath GS, Patel V, Valdiviezo CI, et al. Potentiation of Doxorubicin cardiotoxicity by iron loading in a rodent model. J Am Coll Cardiol 2007;49(25):2457–64.

28. Penel N, Adenis A, Mailliez A, et al. Silent hereditary hematochromatosis as a susceptibility factor of doxorubicin-induced acute cardiac failure. Ann Oncol 2010;21(11):2293–4.

29. Schofield RS, Aranda JM Jr, Hill JA, et al. Cardiac transplantation in a patient with hereditary hemochromatosis: role of adjunctive phlebotomy and erythropoietin. J Heart Lung Transplant 2001;20(6):696–8.

30. Cancado R, Melo MR, de Moraes Bastos R, et al. Deferasirox in patients with iron overload secondary to hereditary hemochromatosis: results of a 1-yr Phase 2 study. Eur J Haematol 2015;95(6):545–50.

31. Lieske JC, Monico CG, Holmes WS, et al. International registry for primary hyperoxaluria. Am J Nephrol 2005;25(3):290–6.

32. Cochat P, Deloraine A, Rotily M, et al. Epidemiology of primary hyperoxaluria type 1. Societe de nephrologie and the societe de nephrologie pediatrique. Nephrol Dial Transplant 1995;10(Suppl 8):3–7.

33. van Woerden CS, Groothoff JW, Wanders RJ, et al. Primary hyperoxaluria type 1 in The Netherlands: prevalence and outcome. Nephrol Dial Transpl 2003;18(2):273–9.

34. Hoppe B. An update on primary hyperoxaluria. Nat Rev Nephrol 2012;8(8):467–75.

35. Salido E, Pey AL, Rodriguez R, et al. Primary hyperoxalurias: disorders of glyoxylate detoxification. Biochim Biophys Acta 2012;1822(9):1453–64.

36. Mookadam F, Smith T, Jiamsripong P, et al. Cardiac abnormalities in primary hyperoxaluria. Circ J 2010;74(11):2403–9.

37. Quan KJ, Biblo LA. Type I primary hyperoxaluria: an unusual presentation of ventricular tachycardia. Cardiol Rev 2003;11(6):318–9.

38. Van Driessche L, Dhondt A, De Sutter J. Heart failure with mitral valve regurgitation due to primary hyperoxaluria type 1: case report with review of the literature. Acta Cardiol 2007;62(2):202–6.

39. Schulze MR, Wachter R, Schmeisser A, et al. Restrictive cardiomyopathy in a patient with primary hyperoxaluria type II. Clin Res Cardiol 2006;95(4):235–40.

40. Detry O, Honore P, DeRoover A, et al. Reversal of oxalosis cardiomyopathy after combined liver and kidney transplantation. Transpl Int 2002;15(1):50–2.

41. Reetz K, Dogan I, Costa AS, et al. Biological and clinical characteristics of the European Friedreich's Ataxia Consortium for Translational Studies (EFACTS) cohort: a cross-sectional analysis of baseline data. Lancet Neurol 2015;14(2):174–82.

42. Schulz JB, Boesch S, Burk K, et al. Diagnosis and treatment of Friedreich ataxia: a European perspective. Nat Rev Neurol 2009;5(4):222–34.

43. Punga T, Buhler M. Long intronic GAA repeats causing Friedreich ataxia impede transcription elongation. EMBO Mol Med 2010;2(4):120–9.

44. Groh M, Lufino MM, Wade-Martins R, et al. R-loops associated with triplet repeat expansions promote gene silencing in Friedreich ataxia and fragile X syndrome. PLoS Genet 2014;10(5):e1004318.

45. Whitnall M, Suryo Rahmanto Y, Huang ML, et al. Identification of nonferritin mitochondrial iron deposits in a mouse model of Friedreich ataxia. Proc Natl Acad Sci U S A 2012;109(50):20590–5.

46. Whitnall M, Suryo Rahmanto Y, Sutak R, et al. The MCK mouse heart model of Friedreich's ataxia: Alterations in iron-regulated proteins and cardiac hypertrophy are limited by iron chelation. Proc Natl Acad Sci United States America 2008;105(28):9757–62.

47. Puccio H, Simon D, Cossee M, et al. Mouse models for Friedreich ataxia exhibit cardiomyopathy, sensory nerve defect and Fe-S enzyme deficiency followed by intramitochondrial iron deposits. Nat Genet 2001;27(2):181–6.

48. Michael S, Petrocine SV, Qian J, et al. Iron and iron-responsive proteins in the cardiomyopathy of Friedreich's ataxia. Cerebellum 2006;5(4):257–67.

49. Campuzano V, Montermini L, Molto MD, et al. Friedreich's ataxia: autosomal recessive disease caused by an intronic GAA triplet repeat expansion. Science 1996;271(5254):1423–7.

50. Cossee M, Puccio H, Gansmuller A, et al. Inactivation of the Friedreich ataxia mouse gene leads to early embryonic lethality without iron accumulation. Hum Mol Genet 2000;9(8):1219–26.

51. Tsou AY, Paulsen EK, Lagedrost SJ, et al. Mortality in Friedreich ataxia. J Neurol Sci 2011;307(1–2):46–9.

52. Regner SR, Lagedrost SJ, Plappert T, et al. Analysis of echocardiograms in a large heterogeneous cohort of patients with friedreich ataxia. Am J Cardiol 2012;109(3):401–5.

53. Evans-Galea MV, Carrodus N, Rowley SM, et al. FXN methylation predicts expression and clinical outcome in Friedreich ataxia. Ann Neurol 2012; 71(4):487–97.

54. McCormick A, Shinnick J, Schadt K, et al. Cardiac transplantation in Friedreich Ataxia: Extended follow-up. J Neurol Sci 2017;375:471–3.

55. Elincx-Benizri S, Glik A, Merkel D, et al. Clinical Experience With Deferiprone Treatment for Friedreich Ataxia. J Child Neurol 2016;31(8):1036–40.

56. Lagedrost SJ, Sutton MS, Cohen MS, et al. Idebenone in Friedreich ataxia cardiomyopathy-results from a 6-month phase III study (IONIA). Am Heart J 2011;161(3):639–45.e1.

57. Tuschl K, Gal A, Paschke E, et al. Mucopolysaccharidosis type II in females: case report and review of literature. Pediatr Neurol 2005;32(4):270–2.

58. Cudry S, Tigaud I, Froissart R, et al. MPS II in females: molecular basis of two different cases. J Med Genet 2000;37(10):E29.

59. Sukegawa K, Matsuzaki T, Fukuda S, et al. Brother/sister siblings affected with Hunter disease: evidence for skewed X chromosome inactivation. Clin Genet 1998;53(2):96–101.

60. Poorthuis BJ, Wevers RA, Kleijer WJ, et al. The frequency of lysosomal storage diseases in The Netherlands. Hum Genet 1999;105(1–2):151–6.

61. Scott CR, Elliott S, Buroker N, et al. Identification of infants at risk for developing Fabry, Pompe, or mucopolysaccharidosis-I from newborn blood spots by tandem mass spectrometry. J Pediatr 2013;163(2):498–503.

62. Braunlin EA, Harmatz PR, Scarpa M, et al. Cardiac disease in patients with mucopolysaccharidosis: presentation, diagnosis and management. J Inherit Metab Dis 2011;34(6):1183–97.

63. Goksel OS, El H, Tireli E, et al. Combined aortic and mitral valve replacement in a child with mucopolysaccharidosis type I: a case report. J Heart Valve Dis 2009;18(2):214–6.

64. Butman SM, Karl L, Copeland JG. Combined aortic and mitral valve replacement in an adult with Scheie's disease. Chest 1989;96(1):209–10.

65. Brands MM, Frohn-Mulder IM, Hagemans ML, et al. Mucopolysaccharidosis: cardiologic features and effects of enzyme-replacement therapy in 24 children with MPS I, II and VI. J Inherit Metab Dis 2013;36(2):227–34.

66. Kampmann C, Lampe C, Whybra-Trumpler C, et al. Mucopolysaccharidosis VI: cardiac involvement and the impact of enzyme replacement therapy. J Inherit Metab Dis 2014;37(2):269–76.

67. Leal GN, de Paula AC, Morhy SS, et al. Advantages of early replacement therapy for mucopolysaccharidosis type VI: echocardiographic follow-up of siblings. Cardiol Young 2014;24(2):229–35.

68. McGill JJ, Inwood AC, Coman DJ, et al. Enzyme replacement therapy for mucopolysaccharidosis VI from 8 weeks of age–a sibling control study. Clin Genet 2010;77(5):492–8.

69. Braunlin E, Rosenfeld H, Kampmann C, et al. Enzyme replacement therapy for mucopolysaccharidosis VI: long-term cardiac effects of galsulfase (Naglazyme®) therapy. J Inherit Metab Dis 2013;36(2):385–94.

70. Giugliani R, Lampe C, Guffon N, et al. Natural history and galsulfase treatment in mucopolysaccharidosis VI (MPS VI, Maroteaux-Lamy syndrome)–10-year follow-up of patients who previously participated in an MPS VI survey study. Am J Med Genet A 2014; 164A(8):1953–64.

71. Elliott PM. Fabry disease: a rare condition emerging from the darkness. Circ Cardiovasc Genet 2017;10(4) [pii:e001862].

72. Germain DP. Fabry disease. Orphanet J Rare Dis 2010;5:30.

73. Echevarria L, Benistan K, Toussaint A, et al. X-chromosome inactivation in female patients with Fabry disease. Clin Genet 2016;89(1):44–54.

74. Lin HY, Chong KW, Hsu JH, et al. High incidence of the cardiac variant of Fabry disease revealed by newborn screening in the Taiwan Chinese population. Circ Cardiovasc Genet 2009;2(5):450–6.

75. Spada M, Pagliardini S, Yasuda M, et al. High incidence of later-onset fabry disease revealed by newborn screening. Am J Hum Genet 2006;79(1): 31–40.

76. Laney DA, Peck DS, Atherton AM, et al. Fabry disease in infancy and early childhood: a systematic literature review. Genet Med 2015;17(5):323–30.

77. Kampmann C, Wiethoff CM, Whybra C, et al. Cardiac manifestations of Anderson-Fabry disease in children and adolescents. Acta Paediatr 2008; 97(4):463–9.

78. Hopkin RJ, Bissler J, Banikazemi M, et al. Characterization of Fabry disease in 352 pediatric patients in the Fabry Registry. Pediatr Res 2008;64(5):550–5.

79. Patel V, O'Mahony C, Hughes D, et al. Clinical and genetic predictors of major cardiac events in patients with Anderson-Fabry disease. Heart 2015; 101(12):961–6.

80. Linhart A, Kampmann C, Zamorano JL, et al. Cardiac manifestations of Anderson-Fabry disease: results from the international Fabry outcome survey. Eur Heart J 2007;28(10):1228–35.

81. Chimenti C, Pieroni M, Morgante E, et al. Prevalence of Fabry disease in female patients with late-onset hypertrophic cardiomyopathy. Circulation 2004;110(9):1047–53.

82. Arends M, Wijburg FA, Wanner C, et al. Favourable effect of early versus late start of enzyme replacement therapy on plasma globotriaosylsphingosine levels in men with classical Fabry disease. Mol Genet Metab 2017;121(2):157–61.

83. Weidemann F, Niemann M, Breunig F, et al. Long-term effects of enzyme replacement therapy on fabry cardiomyopathy: evidence for a better outcome with early treatment. Circulation 2009; 119(4):524–9.

84. Weidemann F, Niemann M, Stork S, et al. Long-term outcome of enzyme-replacement therapy in advanced Fabry disease: evidence for disease progression towards serious complications. J Intern Med 2013;274(4):331–41.

85. Banikazemi M, Bultas J, Waldek S, et al. Agalsidase-beta therapy for advanced Fabry disease: a randomized trial. Ann Intern Med 2007;146(2):77–86.

86. Danon MJ, Oh SJ, DiMauro S, et al. Lysosomal glycogen storage disease with normal acid maltase. Neurology 1981;31(1):51–7.

87. D'Souza RS, Levandowski C, Slavov D, et al. Danon disease: clinical features, evaluation, and management. Circ Heart Fail 2014;7(5):843–9.

88. Rowland TJ, Sweet ME, Mestroni L, et al. Danon disease - dysregulation of autophagy in a multisystem disorder with cardiomyopathy. J Cell Sci 2016;129(11):2135–43.

89. Boucek D, Jirikowic J, Taylor M. Natural history of Danon disease. Genet Med 2011;13(6):563–8.

90. Sugie K, Yamamoto A, Murayama K, et al. Clinicopathological features of genetically confirmed Danon disease. Neurology 2002;58(12):1773–8.

91. Maron BJ, Roberts WC, Arad M, et al. Clinical outcome and phenotypic expression in LAMP2 cardiomyopathy. JAMA 2009;301(12):1253–9.

92. Arad M, Maron BJ, Gorham JM, et al. Glycogen storage diseases presenting as hypertrophic cardiomyopathy. New Engl J Med 2005;352(4):362–72.

93. Singh SR, Zech ATL, Geertz B, et al. Activation of autophagy ameliorates cardiomyopathy in Mybpc3-targeted knockin mice. Circ Heart Fail 2017;10(10) [pii:e004140].

94. Horman S, Beauloye C, Vanoverschelde JL, et al. AMP-activated protein kinase in the control of cardiac metabolism and remodeling. Curr Heart Fail Rep 2012;9(3):164–73.

95. Hinson JT, Chopra A, Lowe A, et al. Integrative Analysis of PRKAG2 Cardiomyopathy iPS and Microtissue Models Identifies AMPK as a Regulator of Metabolism, Survival, and Fibrosis. Cell Rep 2017;19(11):2410.

96. Arad M, Benson DW, Perez-Atayde AR, et al. Constitutively active AMP kinase mutations cause glycogen storage disease mimicking hypertrophic cardiomyopathy. J Clin Invest 2002;109(3):357–62.

97. Gollob MH, Green MS, Tang AS, et al. Identification of a gene responsible for familial Wolff-Parkinson-White syndrome. New Engl J Med 2001;344(24): 1823–31.

98. Mehdirad AA, Fatkin D, DiMarco JP, et al. Electrophysiologic characteristics of accessory atrioventricular connections in an inherited form of Wolff-Parkinson-White syndrome. J Cardiovasc Electrophysiol 1999;10(5):629–35.

99. Porto AG, Brun F, Severini GM, et al. Clinical Spectrum of PRKAG2 Syndrome. Circ Arrhythm Electrophysiol 2016;9(1):e003121.

100. Burwinkel B, Scott JW, Buhrer C, et al. Fatal congenital heart glycogenosis caused by a recurrent activating R531Q mutation in the gamma 2-subunit of AMP-activated protein kinase (PRKAG2), not by phosphorylase kinase deficiency. Am J Hum Genet 2005;76(6):1034–49.

Clinical Presentation and Natural History of Hypertrophic Cardiomyopathy in RASopathies

Giulio Calcagni, MD, PhD[a],*, Rachele Adorisio, MD[a],
Simone Martinelli, PhD[b], Giorgia Grutter, MD[a],
Anwar Baban, MD, PhD[a], Paolo Versacci, MD, PhD[c],
Maria Cristina Digilio, MD[d], Fabrizio Drago, MD[a],
Bruce D. Gelb, MD[e,f], Marco Tartaglia, PhD[d,1],
Bruno Marino, MD[c]

KEYWORDS

- RAS signaling • RASopathies • Noonan syndrome • LEOPARD syndrome • Costello syndrome
- Genotype-phenotype correlations • Congenital heart defect • Hypertrophic cardiomyopathy

KEY POINTS

- RASopathies constitute a family of disorders affecting development and growth caused by dysregulation of intracellular signaling through RAS and the mitogen-activated protein kinase, and PI3K-AKT cascades.
- Hypertrophic cardiomyopathy is a major complication in RASopathies. It is relatively common in Costello syndrome, LEOPARD syndrome, and Noonan syndrome.
- In patients with hypertrophic cardiomyopathy with *PTPN11* and *RAF1* mutations, genotype–phenotype correlation demonstrates upregulation of mitogen-activated protein kinase and PI3K-AKT signaling, underlying hypertrophic cardiomyopathy in RASopathies.
- Congenital heart disease and/or valvular defects are commonly encountered in patients with RASopathy, with or without hypertrophic cardiomyopathy.
- Early onset of hypertrophic cardiomyopathy presenting with cardiac failure have been reported with a worse outcome in patients with RASopathy.

Disclosure statement: B.D. Gelb and M. Tartaglia receive royalties from GeneDx, LabCorp, Prevention Genetics, and Correlegan for genetic testing for Noonan syndrome. All the other authors declare to not have any relationship with a commercial company that has a direct financial interest in subject matter or materials discussed in article or with a company making a competing product.
[a] Department of Pediatric Cardiology and Cardiac Surgery, Bambino Gesù Children's Hospital and Research Institute, Piazza Sant'Onofrio 4, Rome 00165, Italy; [b] Department of Oncology and Molecular Medicine, Istituto Superiore di Sanità, Viale Regina Elena 299, Rome 00161, Italy; [c] Pediatric Cardiology, Department of Pediatrics, Sapienza University, Viale Regina Elena 324, Rome 00161, Italy; [d] Genetics and Rare Diseases Research Division, Bambino Gesù Children's Hospital and Research Institute, Piazza Sant'Onofrio 4, Rome 00165, Italy; [e] Department of Pediatrics, Icahn School of Medicine at Mount Sinai, The Mindich Child Health and Development Institute, One Gustave Levy Place, Box 1042, New York, NY 10029, USA; [f] Department of Genetics and Genomic Sciences, Icahn School of Medicine at Mount Sinai, The Mindich Child Health and Development Institute, One Gustave Levy Place, Box 1042, New York, NY 10029, USA
[1] Present address: Viale di San Paolo, 15, Rome 00146, Italy.
* Corresponding author.
E-mail address: giulio.calcagni@opbg.net

INTRODUCTION

Hypertrophic cardiomyopathy (HCM) is defined by structural and functional abnormalities of the ventricular myocardium leading to increased left ventricular (LV) wall thickness. It was historically subdivided into 2 forms: primary HCM, where no apparent reason is known, and secondary HCM, where an underlying cause can be identified such as valvular, congenital, and systemic disorders.[1] Different studies report a prevalence of unexplained increase in LV thickness in the range of 0.02% to 0.23% in adults; an annual incidence of new cases between 0.24 and 0.47 per 100,000 has been described.[2,3] In the pediatric population, a precise estimation of this condition is lacking; however, preliminary data show that population-based studies report an annual incidence of 0.3 to 0.5 per 100,000.[2,4,5] Recently, HCM was defined by European Society of Cardiology (ESC) by specific morphologic and functional criteria and then classified into familial/genetic and nonfamilial/nongenetic classes.[1] The majority of cases in adult population fall into the familial/genetic category, demonstrating a dominant pattern of inheritance caused by different mutations in cardiac sarcomere genes. In pediatric cohorts, inborn errors of metabolism (glycogen fatty or fatty acid), and neuromuscular, mitochondrial, or lysosomal storage disorders should also be taken in account as an underlying background.[5] A significant subgroup of genetic syndromes has been frequently associated to pediatric HCM, particularly accounting for less than 10% of cases. Of these, Noonan syndrome and related disorders collectively known as RASopathies constitute the most common group of genetic conditions associated with HCM diagnosed in children.[1] Notably, morphologic and clinical features are heterogeneous making complex systematic assessment. Moreover, 20% to 30% of HCM remain elusive to genetic investigations. The aim of this review is to analyze molecular mechanism, clinical presentation, and management of patients with HCM secondary to mutations in the RAS–mitogen-activated protein kinase (RAS-MAPK) pathway genes.

THE RASopathies: CLINICAL FEATURES AND MOLECULAR BASES

Noonan syndrome (MIM 163950) is a clinically variable developmental disorder transmitted as an autosomal-dominant trait, with cardinal features including congenital heart defects (CHDs), HCM, reduced growth, facial dysmorphism, short/webbed neck, ectodermal and skeletal defects, and variable cognitive deficits.[6] Children with Noonan syndrome might be predisposed to a spectrum of hematologic abnormalities and malignancies, depending on the mutated gene and the specific molecular lesion involved.[7] Although Noonan syndrome is a rare disease, it is among the most common nonchromosomal disorders affecting development and growth. In 2001, Tartaglia and coworkers[8] discovered the first Noonan syndrome disease gene, PTPN11, using a positional candidacy approach. Subsequent studies of the same group and others showed that mutations in PTPN11 account for about 50% of cases and established the first clinically relevant genotype–phenotype correlations.[9,10] A subset of germline PTPN11 mutations explain predisposition to myeloproliferative disorders during childhood, whereas a distinct class of somatic lesions in the same gene contribute to childhood leukemia.[11–14] Later work allowed the discovery of 14 additional genes underlying Noonan syndrome or a clinically related traits, namely, KRAS,[15,16] SOS1,[17] RAF1,[18,19] MAP2K1,[20] BRAF,[21] SHOC2,[22] NRAS,[23] CBL,[24,25] RIT1,[26] RRAS,[27] RASA2,[28] LZTR1,[29] SOS2,[29,30] and PPP1CB.[31] These genes occur in approximately 85% to 90% of cases.

There is a group of other rare, autosomal-dominant disorders that are clinically and genetically related to Noonan syndrome. These diseases share dysregulation of RAS signaling as the common pathogenic mechanism and are now collectively named RASopathies.[32,33] Besides the cardiac involvement, major features of RASopathies include defective growth, intellectual disabilities, variable predisposition to pediatric cancers, and ectodermal, muscle and skeletal defects. Among them, Noonan syndrome with multiple lentigines (MIM 151100), formerly LEOPARD syndrome, phenotypically resembles Noonan syndrome, but is specifically characterized by multiple lentigines, sensorineural deafness, and a higher prevalence of HCM and electrocardiographic conduction anomalies. Noonan syndrome with multiple lentigines is allelic with Noonan syndrome, with a restricted spectrum of PTPN11 mutations accounting for the majority of cases, and mutations in RAF1 and BRAF occurring in a small percentage of subjects.[34] Costello syndrome (MIM 218040) and cardiofaciocutaneous syndrome (MIM 115150) exhibit a more severe phenotype compared with Noonan syndrome.[35,36] Whereas the former is genetically homogeneous, being caused by mutations in HRAS, the latter is genetically heterogeneous, with mutations in KRAS, BRAF, MAP2K1, and MAP2K2 accounting for approximately 60% to 80% of cases.[7] RASopathies also includes neurofibromatosis type

1 (MIM 162200), which is caused by inactivating mutations/deletions of the *NF1* gene encoding a RAS-specific GTPase-activating protein[37,38] and Legius syndrome (MIM 611431), caused by inactivating mutations in *SPRED1*,[39] encoding a negative regulator of RAS-mediated RAF1 activation. Overall, the RASopathies are estimated to have an aggregate prevalence of 1:1500 live births.

Based on these discoveries, this family of developmental disorders is now considered as diseases of upregulated RAS-MAPK and PI3K-AKT-mamallian target of rapamycin (mTOR) signaling cascades.[32,40,41] Accordingly, genetic or pharmacologic downregulation of these pathways has been shown to ameliorate developmental features and postnatal issues of RASopathies (eg, growth delay, cardiac defects, HCM, learning deficits, myeloproliferative disease, and neurofibromas).[42–49]

CARDIAC DEFECTS IN RASopathies AND GENOTYPE–PHENOTYPE CORRELATIONS

Several cardiac defects occur in RASopathies with different frequencies among different disorders.[41,50] More than 80% of individuals with Noonan syndrome presents with cardiovascular anomalies, the most common being pulmonary valve stenosis (PVS) for about 50% to 60%, mild-to-severe HCM for 20%, atrioventricular defects (AVCD) and atrial septal defects in less than 10% of patients, and atypical electrocardiographic patterns (approximately 50%).[6] PVS usually shows some typical common features: a dysplastic pulmonary valve, with thickened, elongated, and redundant cusps, as well as supravalvular involvement. This anatomic condition, involving both valvular and supravalvular regions, may explain the frequent unsuccessful percutaneous pulmonary valve treatment by balloon angioplasty,[51,52] resulting in a higher risk of reintervention for this defect. An AVCD is also reported in this subgroup of patients.[53] The partial AVCD form (ostium primum atrial septal defect plus mitral cleft) is more common than complete AVCD.[54] Less frequent CHDs have been reported, including tetralogy of Fallot, patent ductus arteriosus, and left-sided anatomic obstruction at the supravalvular, valvular, or subvalvular level, resulting also in mitral valve (MV) anomalies.[55] Vascular anomalies are rarely associated with RASopathies, mainly aortic dissection,[56] aortic root dilation,[57,58] aneurysm of the sinuses of Valsalva,[59] and coronary arteries dilation.[60] Possible damage owing to RAS-MAPK signal on connective tissue, especially on coronary arteries and aorta, has been proposed, causing coronary arteries wall damage with subsequent ectasia.[60,61]

Excluding CHDs, HCM is the most frequent cardiovascular defect observed in patients affected by RASopathies, and it might represent the major determinant in the outcome of these patients.[62,63] Noonan syndrome-associated HCM arises early in life, with a median age of 5 months.[64,65] The incidence is quite heterogeneous among these syndromes. Approximately 65% of patients with Costello syndrome show HCM, notably higher than for Noonan syndrome, and 40% of them display associated CHDs, including PVS.[66] The most frequent cardiac defect in cardiofaciocutaneous syndrome is PVS, whereas HCM is diagnosed in less than 40% of affected individuals.[67] HCM is also detected in more than 80% of individuals with Noonan syndrome with multiple lentigines, the highest rate among the RASopathies, and tends to occur most commonly during early infancy.[62,68] In addition, these patients display electrocardiographic anomalies (approximately 70%), valvular defects (approximately 50%), PVS (approximately 23%), and coronary arteries defects (approximately 15%). A high percentage of subjects carrying the invariant p.Ser2Gly amino acid substitution in *SHOC2*, which underlie Mazzanti syndrome (also known as Noonan syndrome with loose anagen hair) show cardiac malformations, the most common being septal defects (approximately 42%), PVS (approximately 40%), and MV anomalies (approximately 30%).[22,69] In these patients, the prevalence of HCM is estimated to be about 25%, but its natural history has not been defined as of yet. Cardiac involvement is less common in individuals with neurofibromatosis type 1, Legius syndrome, and Noonan syndrome-like syndrome with *CBL* mutations. **Fig. 1** show the principal heart defect reported in patients with these assorted syndromes according to gene mutation.

Considering the left and right ventricular outflow tract, HCM may occur in obstructive or nonobstructive manner. By convention, LV outflow tract obstructions (LVOTO) is defined as a peak instantaneous Doppler LV outflow tract gradient of 30 mm Hg or greater, but the threshold for invasive treatment is usually considered to be 50 mm Hg or greater. These forms are due to the degree of the hypertrophy, but also to a possible specific role that MV leaflet attachment plays in the mechanism of obstruction.[62] Subaortic stenosis owing to accessory fibrous connective tissue, anomalous insertion of the MV, or to anomalous LV papillary muscles have been frequently reported in patients with syndromic HCM. The length of MV leaflets or the specific attachment of mitral cordae is different in comparison with the MV characteristics in nonsyndromic patients affected by HCM.[70]

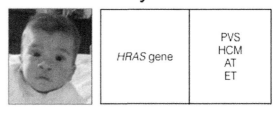

Noonan Syndrome

	PTPN11 gene	PVS (exon 8) ASD (exon 3) AVCD (exons 2,3)
	SOS1 gene	PVS ASD
	RAF1 gene	HCM
	RIT1 gene	PVS HCM
	SHOC2 gene	PVS HCM
	NRAS gene	PVS
	CBL gene	AS MR

Noonan Syndrome with Multiple Lentigines

	PTPN11 gene (Exon 7) (Exon 12) (Exson 13)	HCM Rhythm Distrubances
	RAF1 gene	HCM

CardioFacioCutaneous Syndrome

	BRAF gene	PVS ASD HCM
	MAP2K1 gene MAP2K2 gene	PVS ASD

Costello Syndrome

	HRAS gene	PVS HCM AT ET

Fig. 1. Syndromes, mutated genes, and classical heart defects. AS, aortic stenosis; ASD, atrial septal defect; AT, atrial tachycardia; AVCD, atrioventricular canal defect; ET, ectopic tachycardia; HCM, hypertrophic cardiomyopathy; MR, mitral regurgitation; PVS, pulmonary valve stenosis.

These peculiar anatomic characteristics should be considered carefully before surgical treatment. In patients with Noonan syndrome and symptomatic obstructive HCM, myectomy has been defined as feasible.[51,71] Despite that, the role of MV anomalies as typical marker of complexity in HCM has been previously been associated with a higher risk of reintervention and mortality.[52]

Clinically relevant genotype–phenotype correlations between the cardiac phenotype and both the mutated gene and the specific molecular lesion have been reported. Among patients with Noonan syndrome, PVS is more common (approximately 70%) in subjects with PTPN11 and SOS1 mutations, and it is less common (approximately 20%) in patients with RAF1 lesions.[9,18,72] In contrast,

HCM prevalence is relatively low in patients harboring Noonan syndrome-causing *PTPN11* or *SOS1* mutations, but it is overrepresented in *RAF1*-associated Noonan syndrome (approximately 75%), where it seems to be allele specific; it is associated with mutations affecting the *N*-terminal 14-3-3 consensus motif or the *C*-terminus of the protein.[18,32] Furthermore, a different class of *RAF1* mutations has recently been identified in nonsyndromic, childhood-onset dilated cardiomyopathy.[73] Of note, mutation-specific associations have been identified also for *PTPN11*, with a distinct class of mutations underlying Noonan syndrome with multiple lentigines specifically associated with a higher prevalence of HCM.[62,63] Finally, compared with the general Noonan syndrome population, the prevalence and severity of both HCM and CHD seem to be relatively high in patients carrying heterozygous *RIT1* mutations.[26,74]

MOLECULAR MECHANISMS OF HYPERTROPHIC CARDIOMYOPATHY IN RASopathies

The molecular pathogenesis of HCM in RASopathies results from hyperactivation of different signaling pathways. Increased signaling through the RAS-MAPK cascade was demonstrated in multiple cell types, including cardiac fibroblasts and neonatal cardiomyocytes of a mouse model of Noonan syndrome bearing the p.Leu613Val mutation in the *Raf1* gene.[75] Consistent with this evidence, treatment with a MEK inhibitor rescued the cardiac phenotype of Raf1[L613V/+] mice. In contrast, increased signal flow through the PI3K-AKT-mTOR pathway has been reported in cardiomyocytes from a mouse model of Noonan syndrome with multiple lentigines bearing the p.Tyr279Cys mutation in the *Ptpn11* gene, whereas ligand-evoked Erk phosphorylation was documented to be impaired in these mice.[49] Treatment of the *Ptpn11*[Y279C/+] mice with rapamycin, an mTOR inhibitor, or with the AKT inhibitor ARQ092, normalized HCM.[49,76] These findings were consistent with previous data, indicating a positive role of Noonan syndrome with multiple lentigines–associated *PTPN11* mutants on AKT activation.[40] Similarly, *RAF1* mutations causing nonsyndromic dilated cardiomyopathy were shown to cause BRAF-dependent AKT hyperactivation, suggesting possible therapeutic efficacy of mTOR inhibitors.[73] Remarkably, short-term therapy with an mTOR inhibitor, namely, everolimus, has recently been used to prevent congestive heart failure (CHF) in a patients with Noonan syndrome with multiple lentigines with a severe form of HCM, even though no reversal of cardiac hypertrophy was noted.[77]

CLINICAL CHARACTERISTICS OF HYPERTROPHIC CARDIOMYOPATHY IN RASopathies

HCM in RASopathies is characterized by asymmetrical hypertrophy with major involvement of basal interventricular septum. Other myocardial regions, such as the apex, the midportion, and the posterior wall of the LV, might also be involved. According to the ESC guidelines, adult LV wall thickness of greater than 15 mm is considered as the gold standard for diagnosis.[1] Genetic and nongenetic disorders can present with minor degrees of wall thickening (13–14 mm); in these selected conditions, the diagnosis of HCM requires evaluation of other features, including family history, noncardiac symptoms and signs, electrocardiographic changes, laboratory investigations, and multimodality cardiac imaging. In children, the diagnosis requires a segmental LV wall thickness more than 2 standard deviations greater than the predicted mean for age, sex, and height–weight ratio.[1] The hypertrophy is usually nonspecific and asymmetrical with the ratio of the thickness of the septum to the free wall of the LV of greater than 1.3 to 1.0. Compared with other types of HCM, those associated with the RASopathies show more ventricular hypertrophy and an increased prevalence of LVOTO. These patients usually have a higher grade of right ventricular hypertrophy.[78]

Other morphologic features characterize the RASopathies group HCM in a unique fashion. Structural abnormalities such as elongation of MV with an anomalous insertion,[55] and abnormal displacement of papillary muscles have been described.[79] Congenital anomalies of the pulmonary valve are frequently encountered in this subgroup. Usually in Noonan syndrome, severe HCM presents early in life, and these patients are at greatest risk of long-term morbidities,[80] suggesting a tailored management according to the etiology of the HCM. In this subgroup of patients, severe PVS is often associated with HCM. Dilated coronary arteries are reported in the context of HCM owing to RAS-MAPK mutations, irrespective of the grade of HCM.

Owing to the higher degree of hypertrophy and the associated valvular abnormalities, several pathophysiologic features should be addressed during clinical evaluation, including diastolic dysfunction, LVOTO, myocardial ischemia, and cardiac arrhythmias.

Diastolic dysfunction is quite common in HCM and occurs owing to both abnormal relaxation and reduced ventricular compliance.[78] It usually manifests as exertional dyspnea and exercise intolerance since infancy. Of course, for this early age group, feeding difficulties and failure to thrive are the most pronounced symptoms. As mentioned,[78] the Noonan syndrome group is characterized by both marked HCM and diastolic dysfunction (**Fig. 2**). These morphologic and functional findings could explain the different symptoms and clinical events in this subgroup, and potentially define the more appropriate therapeutic options in children with HCM of different etiology. In addition, LVOTO should be addressed during a routine evaluation. This pattern is often associated to systolic anterior movement[62] of the MV or to midcavitary LV obstruction. The outflow obstruction is worsened by exercise. The RASopathy subgroup, mainly in the context of Noonan syndrome, usually shows a more severe pattern of LVOTO.[78]

Myocardial ischemia is common among patients with HCM, including young adolescents with RASopathies. These symptoms are due to reduced myocardial perfusion through the increased myocardial mass. Coronary arteries abnormalities (dilation of main left coronary artery, anterior descending artery, or right coronary arteries) have been reported in RASopathies patients associated with HCM.[62] These features, which could occur also in the setting of CHDs independent from the specific genetic change, could also explain the higher risk of myocardial ischemia in these patients.

Other frequent manifestations of HCM in RASopathies are arrhythmias. Supraventricular and ventricular ectopic beats are common, and nonsustained ventricular tachycardia is frequent and related to the risk for sudden cardiac death. The current ESC guidelines provide different factors for assessing the risk of sudden cardiac death.[1] In children, LV wall thickness of more than 6 standard deviations and/or a previous history of life-threatening arrhythmias[81,82] are current indications for implantable cardioverter-defibrillator implantation. In the pediatric population, other specific risk factors include CHF,[83] increased LV posterior wall thickness,[84] and the presence of coronary myocardial bridging.[85] However, there is no specific risk score tool for the estimation of sudden cardiac death in children to date.

Almost 25% of patients with HCM die because of CHF in the first year of life, although the rate of sudden death is lower, compared with that reported in familial HCM.[86] Adult patients with Noonan syndrome and HCM are also predisposed to develop dilated cardiomyopathy.[87]

IMPLICATIONS FOR TREATMENT: FROM MEDICAL MANAGEMENT TO SURGICAL TREATMENT

Clinical management is based on a tailored approach according to the specific phenotype including symptoms, arrhythmias, the degree of hypertrophy, and LVOTO.

In the subgroup of patients with Noonan syndrome with HCM, outcomes are worse in infants compared with older children. In patients with HCM and Noonan syndrome, a more severe cardiac involvement correlate with a lower survival rate,[65] supporting the hypothesis that HCM in Noonan syndrome, is an important risk factor for death. Significant diastolic dysfunction has been advocated as the principal cause. Moreover, in the Noonan syndrome subgroup, children with CHF in the first 6 months of life have been demonstrated to have a lower survival rate compared with their peers without CHF.[65] These data have been recently confirmed in a study reporting a higher risk for mortality in those younger than

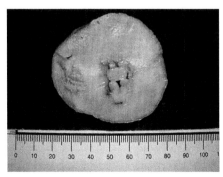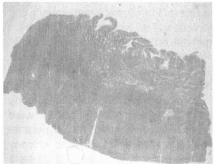

Fig. 2. Anatomic and histologic specimen of left ventricle hypertrophy. *Left,* Anatomic specimen: short axis left ventricle in a patient with hypertrophic cardiomyopathy and Noonan syndrome with multiple lentigines. *Right,* Histologic specimen of left ventricle wall (hematoxylin-eosin, original magnification × 1.25). (*Courtesy of* Paola Francalanci, MD, Rome, Italy.)

2 years old or in adolescents.[52] In particular, low cardiac output, next to surgical treatment for CHD or HCM, was reported in the subgroup of patient who died for cardiac causes.[52]

Throughout the lifespan of patients with Costello syndrome, specific cardiac follow-up for HCM is required, especially in the first 2 years of life. The frequency of screening depends on the severity of hypertrophy. Annual evaluation and risk stratification at puberty are mandatory in the Costello syndrome subgroup.[66] Medical management includes periodic evaluation in asymptomatic patients.

Medical therapy is the first-line option in the treatment of the majority of patients with RASopathies. General guidelines are followed here for treatment. Drugs such as beta-blockers, dysopiramide, and L-type calcium channel blockers are used in the treatment of patients with HCM to reduce symptoms and the degree of obstruction.[88] Beta-blockers are the first-line management in HCM using nonvasodilating beta-blockers titrated to the maximum tolerated dose. Dysopiramide is also indicated when added to beta-blockers, reducing the degree of obstruction. Finally, calcium channel blockers are effective when patients are not responding to beta-blockers. In cases of CHF, diuretics may be indicated, counterbalancing the effect on hypotension, and LVOTO.[1]

Surgical myectomy is the treatment of choice when patients seem to be symptomatic for severe LVOTO, despite maximal therapy.[89,90] Children with RASopathies and LVOTO show earlier cardiac symptoms compared with nonsyndromic HCM. In addition, greater mortality is reported in symptomatic children with LVOTO and Noonan syndrome compared with nonsyndromic HCM. Therefore, some centers advocate an early cardiac transplantation for selected patients not eligible for surgery.[65] Surgical relief of LVOTO in specialized centers with experience in pediatric surgical myectomy has been considered a practical alternative to transplantation.[71]

Orthotropic heart transplantation is rarely reported for patients with HCM and RASopathy syndrome.[86] It should be considered in eligible patients who have an LV ejection fraction of less than 50% and a New York Heart Association functional class of III to IV symptoms despite an optimal anti-CHF treatment, intractable ventricular arrhythmia, or severe diastolic dysfunction (even in case of normal ejection fraction).[1] Orthotropic heart transplantation has also been used as a life-saving strategy for some HCM patients, but the risk factors and outcomes have not been scrutinized scientifically. However, rejection has been reported as a cause of death after heart transplantation.[52]

Looking after patients on the waiting list for heart transplantation and taking into account the cumulative mortality risk (during the waiting list time or after transplantation), some authors described that United Network for Organ Sharing status 1 and age less than 1 year at the time of listing were associated with poorer outcomes compared status 2 and older status 1.[91] No specific data have been reported with respect to phenotype and genotype RAS-MAPK cascade vis-á-vis eligibility for heart transplantation, but an accurate analysis of all additional risk factors should be considered carefully to better define the timing of listing and which patient subgroup may derive optimal benefit from a heart transplant.[91] Cumulative wait list mortality, consistent with the Pediatric Cardiomyopathy Registry and Australian Registry, was significantly higher (within 2–3 months after listing). This finding is higher in infants with HCM[3,4] and suggests a more malignant natural history for the infantile form compared with HCM presenting later. The high mortality rate after orthotropic heart transplantation may also be related to morbidities in high-priority, critically ill infants. For these reasons, orthotropic heart transplantation in RASopathies should be considered as early as possible and before clinical deterioration, especially given the good outcomes after successful heart transplantation.[91]

SUMMARY

RASopathies constitute a family of disorders affecting development and growth caused by dysregulation of intracellular signaling through RAS and the MAPK, and PI3K-AKT cascades. HCM, with or without congenital heart disease, is common and represents a major complication in these patients. Surgical treatment, despite medical therapy, can be an option, even though a worse outcome has been described for patients with RASopathies presenting with an early onset of HCM and cardiac failure.

Upregulation of MAPK and PI3K-AKT has been described in patients with HCM with *PTPN11* and *RAF1* mutations, suggesting that a short-term mTOR inhibitor therapy could be useful to prevent heart failure in patients with a severe form of HCM.

ACKNOWLEDGMENTS

The authors thank Dr Paola Francalanci, MD, for **Fig. 2**, Dr Elena Pelliccione, C.C.P., for her technical assistance, and Dr Elisa Del Vecchio for her valuable collaboration in the editorial revision.

REFERENCES

1. Authors/Task Force Members, Elliott PM, Anastasakis A, Borger MA, et al. 2014 ESC guidelines on diagnosis and management of hypertrophic cardiomyopathy: the task force for the diagnosis and management of hypertrophic cardiomyopathy of the European society of cardiology (ESC). Eur Heart J 2014;35(39):2733–79.
2. Lipshultz SE, Sleeper LA, Towbin JA, et al. The incidence of pediatric cardiomyopathy in two regions of the United States. N Engl J Med 2003;348(17): 1647–55.
3. Colan SD, Lipshultz SE, Lowe AM, et al. Epidemiology and cause-specific outcome of hypertrophic cardiomyopathy in children: findings from the pediatric cardiomyopathy registry. Circulation 2007; 115(6):773–81.
4. Nugent AW, Daubeney PE, Chondros P, et al. Clinical features and outcomes of childhood hypertrophic cardiomyopathy: results from a national population-based study. Circulation 2005;112(9): 1332–8.
5. Moak JP, Kaski JP. Hypertrophic cardiomyopathy in children. Heart 2012;98(14):1044–54.
6. Roberts AE, Allanson JE, Tartaglia M, et al. Noonan syndrome. Lancet 2013;381(9863):333–42.
7. Tartaglia M, Gelb BD, Zenker M. Noonan syndrome and clinically related disorders. Best Pract Res Clin Endocrinol Metab 2011;25(1):161–79.
8. Tartaglia M, Mehler EL, Goldberg R, et al. Mutations in PTPN11, encoding the protein tyrosine phosphatase SHP-2, cause Noonan syndrome. Nat Genet 2001;29(4):465–8.
9. Tartaglia M, Kalidas K, Shaw A, et al. PTPN11 mutations in Noonan syndrome: molecular spectrum, genotype-phenotype correlation, and phenotypic heterogeneity. Am J Hum Genet 2002;70(6): 1555–63.
10. Zenker M, Buheitel G, Rauch R, et al. Genotype-phenotype correlations in Noonan syndrome. J Pediatr 2004;144(3):368–74.
11. Tartaglia M, Niemeyer CM, Fragale A, et al. Somatic mutations in PTPN11 in juvenile myelomonocytic leukemia, myelodysplastic syndromes and acute myeloid leukemia. Nat Genet 2003;34(2):148–50.
12. Tartaglia M, Martinelli S, Cazzaniga G, et al. Genetic evidence for lineage-related and differentiation stage-related contribution of somatic PTPN11 mutations to leukemogenesis in childhood acute leukemia. Blood 2004;104(2):307–13.
13. Tartaglia M, Martinelli S, Stella L, et al. Diversity and functional consequences of germline and somatic PTPN11 mutations in human disease. Am J Hum Genet 2006;78(2):279–90.
14. Strullu M, Caye A, Lachenaud J, et al. Juvenile myelomonocytic leukaemia and Noonan syndrome. J Med Genet 2014;51(10):689–97.
15. Carta C, Pantaleoni F, Bocchinfuso G, et al. Germline missense mutations affecting KRAS isoform B are associated with a severe Noonan syndrome phenotype. Am J Hum Genet 2006;79(1):129–35.
16. Schubbert S, Zenker M, Rowe SL, et al. Germline KRAS mutations cause Noonan syndrome. Nat Genet 2006;38(3):331–6.
17. Tartaglia M, Pennacchio LA, Zhao C, et al. Gain-of-function SOS1 mutations cause a distinctive form of Noonan syndrome. Nat Genet 2007;39(1):75–9.
18. Pandit B, Sarkozy A, Pennacchio LA, et al. Gain-of-function RAF1 mutations cause Noonan and LEOPARD syndromes with hypertrophic cardiomyopathy. Nat Genet 2007;39(8):1007–12.
19. Razzaque MA, Nishizawa T, Komoike Y, et al. Germline gain-of-function mutations in RAF1 cause Noonan syndrome. Nat Genet 2007;39(8):1013–7.
20. Nava C, Hanna N, Michot C, et al. Cardio-facio-cutaneous and Noonan syndromes due to mutations in the RAS/MAPK signalling pathway: genotype-phenotype relationships and overlap with Costello syndrome. J Med Genet 2007;44(12):763–71.
21. Sarkozy A, Carta C, Moretti S, et al. Germline BRAF mutations in Noonan, LEOPARD, and cardiofaciocutaneous syndromes: molecular diversity and associated phenotypic spectrum. Hum Mutat 2009;30(4): 695–702.
22. Cordeddu V, Di Schiavi E, Pennacchio LA, et al. Mutation of SHOC2 promotes aberrant protein N-myristoylation and causes noonan-like syndrome with loose anagen hair. Nat Genet 2009;41(9):1022–6.
23. Cirstea IC, Kutsche K, Dvorsky R, et al. A restricted spectrum of NRAS mutations causes Noonan syndrome. Nat Genet 2010;42(1):27–9.
24. Martinelli S, De Luca A, Stellacci E, et al. Heterozygous germline mutations in the CBL tumor-suppressor gene cause a Noonan syndrome-like phenotype. Am J Hum Genet 2010;87(2):250–7.
25. Perez B, Mechinaud F, Galambrun C, et al. Germline mutations of the CBL gene define a new genetic syndrome with predisposition to juvenile myelomonocytic leukaemia. J Med Genet 2010;47(10):686–91.
26. Aoki Y, Niihori T, Banjo T, et al. Gain-of-function mutations in RIT1 cause Noonan syndrome, a RAS/MAPK pathway syndrome. Am J Hum Genet 2013; 93(1):173–80.
27. Flex E, Jaiswal M, Pantaleoni F, et al. Activating mutations in RRAS underlie a phenotype within the RASopathy spectrum and contribute to leukaemogenesis. Hum Mol Genet 2014;23(16): 4315–27.

28. Chen PC, Yin J, Yu HW, et al. Next-generation sequencing identifies rare variants associated with Noonan syndrome. Proc Natl Acad Sci U S A 2014;111(31):11473–8.

29. Yamamoto GL, Aguena M, Gos M, et al. Rare variants in SOS2 and LZTR1 are associated with Noonan syndrome. J Med Genet 2015;52(6):413–21.

30. Cordeddu V, Yin JC, Gunnarsson C, et al. Activating mutations affecting the dbl homology domain of SOS2 cause Noonan syndrome. Hum Mutat 2015; 36(11):1080–7.

31. Gripp KW, Aldinger KA, Bennett JT, et al. A novel rasopathy caused by recurrent de novo missense mutations in PPP1CB closely resembles Noonan syndrome with loose anagen hair. Am J Med Genet A 2016;170(9):2237–47.

32. Tartaglia M, Gelb BD. Disorders of dysregulated signal traffic through the RAS-MAPK pathway: phenotypic spectrum and molecular mechanisms. Ann N Y Acad Sci 2010;1214:99–121.

33. Rauen KA. The RASopathies. Annu Rev Genomics Hum Genet 2013;14:355–69.

34. Sarkozy A, Digilio MC, Dallapiccola B. Leopard syndrome. Orphanet J Rare Dis 2008;3:13.

35. Roberts A, Allanson J, Jadico SK, et al. The cardiofaciocutaneous syndrome. J Med Genet 2006; 43(11):833–42.

36. Gripp KW, Lin AE. Costello syndrome: a ras/mitogen activated protein kinase pathway syndrome (rasopathy) resulting from HRAS germline mutations. Genet Med 2012;14(3):285–92.

37. Klose A, Ahmadian MR, Schuelke M, et al. Selective disactivation of neurofibromin GAP activity in neurofibromatosis type 1. Hum Mol Genet 1998;7(8): 1261–8.

38. Pasmant E, Vidaud M, Vidaud D, et al. Neurofibromatosis type 1: from genotype to phenotype. J Med Genet 2012;49(8):483–9.

39. Brems H, Chmara M, Sahbatou M, et al. Germline loss-of-function mutations in SPRED1 cause a neurofibromatosis 1-like phenotype. Nat Genet 2007;39(9):1120–6.

40. Edouard T, Combier JP, Nedelec A, et al. Functional effects of PTPN11 (SHP2) mutations causing LEOPARD syndrome on epidermal growth factor-induced phosphoinositide 3-kinase/AKT/glycogen synthase kinase 3beta signaling. Mol Cell Biol 2010;30(10): 2498–507.

41. Aoki Y, Niihori T, Inoue S, et al. Recent advances in RASopathies. J Hum Genet 2016;61(1):33–9.

42. Nakamura T, Colbert M, Krenz M, et al. Mediating ERK 1/2 signaling rescues congenital heart defects in a mouse model of Noonan syndrome. J Clin Invest 2007;117(8):2123–32.

43. Krenz M, Gulick J, Osinska HE, et al. Role of ERK1/2 signaling in congenital valve malformations in Noonan syndrome. Proc Natl Acad Sci U S A 2008;105(48):18930–5.

44. Araki T, Chan G, Newbigging S, et al. Noonan syndrome cardiac defects are caused by PTPN11 acting in endocardium to enhance endocardial-mesenchymal transformation. Proc Natl Acad Sci U S A 2009;106(12):4736–41.

45. Chen PC, Wakimoto H, Conner D, et al. Activation of multiple signaling pathways causes developmental defects in mice with a Noonan syndrome-associated Sos1 mutation. J Clin Invest 2010; 120(12):4353–65.

46. De Rocca Serra-Nedelec A, Edouard T, Treguer K, et al. Noonan syndrome-causing SHP2 mutants inhibit insulin-like growth factor 1 release via growth hormone-induced ERK hyperactivation, which contributes to short stature. Proc Natl Acad Sci U S A 2012;109(11):4257–62.

47. Jessen WJ, Miller SJ, Jousma E, et al. MEK inhibition exhibits efficacy in human and mouse neurofibromatosis tumors. J Clin Invest 2013; 123(1):340–7.

48. Schramm C, Edwards MA, Krenz M. New approaches to prevent LEOPARD syndrome-associated cardiac hypertrophy by specifically targeting Shp2-dependent signaling. J Biol Chem 2013;288(25):18335–44.

49. Marin TM, Keith K, Davies B, et al. Rapamycin reverses hypertrophic cardiomyopathy in a mouse model of LEOPARD syndrome-associated PTPN11 mutation. J Clin Invest 2011;121(3):1026–43.

50. Gelb BD, Roberts AE, Tartaglia M. Cardiomyopathies in Noonan syndrome and the other RASopathies. Prog Pediatr Cardiol 2015;39(1):13–9.

51. Prendiville TW, Gauvreau K, Tworog-Dube E, et al. Cardiovascular disease in Noonan syndrome. Arch Dis Child 2014;99(7):629–34.

52. Calcagni G, Limongelli G, D'Ambrosio A, et al. Cardiac defects, morbidity and mortality in patients affected by RASopathies. CARNET study results. Int J Cardiol 2017;245:92–8.

53. Marino B, Digilio MC, Toscano A, et al. Congenital heart diseases in children with Noonan syndrome: an expanded cardiac spectrum with high prevalence of atrioventricular canal. J Pediatr 1999; 135(6):703–6.

54. Marino B, Digilio MC, Gagliardi MG, et al. Partial atrioventricular canal with left-sided obstruction in patients with Noonan syndrome. Pediatr Cardiol 1996;17(4):278.

55. Marino B, Gagliardi MG, Digilio MC, et al. Noonan syndrome: structural abnormalities of the mitral valve causing subaortic obstruction. Eur J Pediatr 1995;154(12):949–52.

56. Shachter N, Perloff JK, Mulder DG. Aortic dissection in Noonan's syndrome (46 XY turner). Am J Cardiol 1984;54(3):464–5.

57. Power PD, Lewin MB, Hannibal MC, et al. Aortic root dilatation is a rare complication of Noonan syndrome. Pediatr Cardiol 2006;27(4):478–80.

58. Cornwall JW, Green RS, Nielsen JC, et al. Frequency of aortic dilation in Noonan syndrome. Am J Cardiol 2014;113(2):368–71.

59. Purnell R, Williams I, Von Oppell U, et al. Giant aneurysms of the sinuses of Valsalva and aortic regurgitation in a patient with Noonan's syndrome. Eur J Cardiothorac Surg 2005;28(2):346–8.

60. Calcagni G, Baban A, De Luca E, et al. Coronary artery ectasia in Noonan syndrome: report of an individual with SOS1 mutation and literature review. Am J Med Genet A 2016;170(3):665–9.

61. Ucar T, Atalay S, Tekin M, et al. Bilateral coronary artery dilatation and supravalvular pulmonary stenosis in a child with Noonan syndrome. Pediatr Cardiol 2005;26(6):848–50.

62. Limongelli G, Pacileo G, Marino B, et al. Prevalence and clinical significance of cardiovascular abnormalities in patients with the LEOPARD syndrome. Am J Cardiol 2007;100(4):736–41.

63. Limongelli G, Sarkozy A, Pacileo G, et al. Genotype-phenotype analysis and natural history of left ventricular hypertrophy in LEOPARD syndrome. Am J Med Genet A 2008;146A(5):620–8.

64. Hickey EJ, Mehta R, Elmi M, et al. Survival implications: hypertrophic cardiomyopathy in Noonan syndrome. Congenit Heart Dis 2011;6(1):41–7.

65. Wilkinson JD, Lowe AM, Salbert BA, et al. Outcomes in children with Noonan syndrome and hypertrophic cardiomyopathy: a study from the pediatric cardiomyopathy registry. Am Heart J 2012;164(3):442–8.

66. Lin AE, Alexander ME, Colan SD, et al. Clinical, pathological, and molecular analyses of cardiovascular abnormalities in Costello syndrome: a ras/MAPK pathway syndrome. Am J Med Genet A 2011;155A(3):486–507.

67. Allanson JE, Anneren G, Aoki Y, et al. Cardio-facio-cutaneous syndrome: does genotype predict phenotype? Am J Med Genet C Semin Med Genet 2011;157C(2):129–35.

68. Lauriol J, Kontaridis MI. PTPN11-associated mutations in the heart: has LEOPARD changed its RASpots? Trends Cardiovasc Med 2011;21(4):97–104.

69. Komatsuzaki S, Aoki Y, Niihori T, et al. Mutation analysis of the SHOC2 gene in noonan-like syndrome and in hematologic malignancies. J Hum Genet 2010;55(12):801–9.

70. Maron MS, Olivotto I, Harrigan C, et al. Mitral valve abnormalities identified by cardiovascular magnetic resonance represent a primary phenotypic expression of hypertrophic cardiomyopathy. Circulation 2011;124(1):40–7.

71. Poterucha JT, Johnson JN, O'Leary PW, et al. Surgical ventricular septal myectomy for patients with Noonan syndrome and symptomatic left ventricular outflow tract obstruction. Am J Cardiol 2015;116(7):1116–21.

72. Lepri F, De Luca A, Stella L, et al. SOS1 mutations in Noonan syndrome: molecular spectrum, structural insights on pathogenic effects, and genotype-phenotype correlations. Hum Mutat 2011;32(7):760–72.

73. Dhandapany PS, Razzaque MA, Muthusami U, et al. RAF1 mutations in childhood-onset dilated cardiomyopathy. Nat Genet 2014;46(6):635–9.

74. Calcagni G, Baban A, Lepri FR, et al. Congenital heart defects in Noonan syndrome and RIT1 mutation. Genet Med 2016;18(12):1320.

75. Wu X, Simpson J, Hong JH, et al. MEK-ERK pathway modulation ameliorates disease phenotypes in a mouse model of Noonan syndrome associated with the Raf1(L613V) mutation. J Clin Invest 2011;121(3):1009–25.

76. Wang J, Chandrasekhar V, Abbadessa G, et al. In vivo efficacy of the AKT inhibitor ARQ 092 in Noonan syndrome with multiple lentigines-associated hypertrophic cardiomyopathy. PLoS One 2017;12(6):e0178905.

77. Hahn A, Lauriol J, Thul J, et al. Rapidly progressive hypertrophic cardiomyopathy in an infant with Noonan syndrome with multiple lentigines: palliative treatment with a rapamycin analog. Am J Med Genet A 2015;167A(4):744–51.

78. Cerrato F, Pacileo G, Limongelli G, et al. A standard echocardiographic and tissue doppler study of morphological and functional findings in children with hypertrophic cardiomyopathy compared to those with left ventricular hypertrophy in the setting of Noonan and LEOPARD syndromes. Cardiol Young 2008;18(6):575–80.

79. Hirsch HD, Gelband H, Garcia O, et al. Rapidly progressive obstructive cardiomyopathy in infants with Noonan's syndrome. Report of two cases. Circulation 1975;52(6):1161–5.

80. Colquitt JL, Noonan JA. Cardiac findings in Noonan syndrome on long-term follow-up. Congenit Heart Dis 2014;9(2):144–50.

81. Limongelli G, Pacileo G, Calabro R. Is sudden cardiac death predictable in LEOPARD syndrome? Cardiol Young 2006;16(6):599–601.

82. Priori SG, Blomstrom-Lundqvist C, Mazzanti A, et al. 2015 ESC guidelines for the management of patients with ventricular arrhythmias and the prevention of sudden cardiac death: the Task Force for the Management of Patients with Ventricular Arrhythmias and the Prevention of Sudden Cardiac Death of the European Society of Cardiology (ESC). Endorsed by: Association for European Paediatric

and Congenital Cardiology (AEPC). Eur Heart J 2015;36(41):2793–867.

83. Maron BJ, Tajik AJ, Ruttenberg HD, et al. Hypertrophic cardiomyopathy in infants: clinical features and natural history. Circulation 1982;65(1):7–17.

84. Suda K, Kohl T, Kovalchin JP, et al. Echocardiographic predictors of poor outcome in infants with hypertrophic cardiomyopathy. Am J Cardiol 1997;80(5):595–600.

85. Yetman AT, McCrindle BW, MacDonald C, et al. Myocardial bridging in children with hypertrophic cardiomyopathy–a risk factor for sudden death. N Engl J Med 1998;339(17):1201–9.

86. Shaw AC, Kalidas K, Crosby AH, et al. The natural history of Noonan syndrome: a long-term follow-up study. Arch Dis Child 2007;92(2):128–32.

87. Pierpont ME, Magoulas PL, Adi S, et al. Cardio-facio-cutaneous syndrome: clinical features, diagnosis, and management guidelines. Pediatrics 2014;134(4):e1149–62.

88. Ostman-Smith I. Beta-blockers in pediatric hypertrophic cardiomyopathies. Rev Recent Clin Trials 2014; 9(2):82–5.

89. Minakata K, Dearani JA, O'Leary PW, et al. Septal myectomy for obstructive hypertrophic cardiomyopathy in pediatric patients: early and late results. Ann Thorac Surg 2005;80(4):1424–9 [discussion: 1429–30].

90. Hickey EJ, McCrindle BW, Larsen SH, et al. Hypertrophic cardiomyopathy in childhood: disease natural history, impact of obstruction, and its influence on survival. Ann Thorac Surg 2012;93(3):840–8.

91. Gajarski R, Naftel DC, Pahl E, et al. Outcomes of pediatric patients with hypertrophic cardiomyopathy listed for transplant. J Heart Lung Transplant 2009; 28(12):1329–34.

Moving?

Make sure your subscription moves with you!

To notify us of your new address, find your **Clinics Account Number** (located on your mailing label above your name), and contact customer service at:

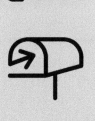

Email: journalscustomerservice-usa@elsevier.com

800-654-2452 (subscribers in the U.S. & Canada)
314-447-8871 (subscribers outside of the U.S. & Canada)

Fax number: 314-447-8029

Elsevier Health Sciences Division
Subscription Customer Service
3251 Riverport Lane
Maryland Heights, MO 63043

*To ensure uninterrupted delivery of your subscription, please notify us at least 4 weeks in advance of move.

Printed and bound by CPI Group (UK) Ltd, Croydon, CR0 4YY

03/10/2024

01040382-0020